Loving Your Body

Loving Your Body

KEN KEYES, JR.

Living Love Publications
c/o Cornucopia Institute
St. Mary, Kentucky 40063

Copyright © 1974 by Ken Keyes, Jr.
Library of Congress Catalog Card Number: 74-84411.
International Standard Book Number: 0-9600688-4-8.

This book was originally published under the title, *How to Live Longer-Stronger-Slimmer*, by Frederick Fell, Inc., New York, New York and was copyrighted in 1966 by Kenneth S. Keyes, Jr.

LIVING LOVE PUBLICATIONS
c/o CORNUCOPIA INSTITUTE
St. Mary, KY 40063

*This book is dedicated
to those who deeply embrace
the world with their hearts;
who accept themselves and
therefore give freedom to others;
who love themselves and
thereby love all others —
without conditions,
without demands,
without expectations.*

ACKNOWLEDGMENTS

First of all, I wish to acknowledge my great debt to Dr. William A. McCall of Teachers College, Columbia, New York City, for the inspiration, encouragement, and assistance he has given me for over two decades. My association with this outstanding scientist has meant more to me than words can express.

I especially wish to thank Dr. Faye Grant of the University of Miami for the countless ways she has helped me in my study in the field of nutrition. I am indebted to her for many helpful suggestions both for the manuscript and the Food Table. Since this book explores the area beyond academic nutrition, I alone have the full responsibility for all errors of omission or commission.

I wish to record my thanks to Mona Fredericks, Doris Kaufmann, Patricia Kimball, Elizabeth Larsen, Dr. and Mrs. William McCall, Henry Raepple, Barbara Rasmussen, Deedee Roberts, and my mother, Lucille Evans, who have given me the benefit of their reactions to the manuscript. Many thanks are due to Marion Kley for her editorial assistance. I also want to express my appreciation to Beverly Robinson for her help in preparing the Food Table. Doris Pinson deserves much credit for her intelligent typing of the manuscript. I wish to thank especially

Gerda E. Voyes of the Science Library of the University of Miami for her willing cooperation in furnishing me with materials required for the extensive research upon which this book has been based. My appreciation also goes to Dr. C. E. Bild for the generous use of books from his professional library. Bonita Keyes has generously relieved me of the task of proofreading. Thanks are due to Mrs. Velma Richards for her excellent suggestions. And last, but not least, I wish to express my appreciation to Mrs. LaRue Storm for first directing my attention to the fascinating study of nutrition.

I also am grateful to the authors and publishers who have given permission to quote from their publications.

KENNETH S. KEYES, JR.

Coconut Grove, Florida

CONTENTS

Nutrition is everyone's adventure.
We can and should both *add life to*
our years and *add years to our lives.*

Dr. Henry C. Sherman
Columbia University

FOREWORD

A knowledge of nutrition is essential if we wish to enjoy our bodies to the fullest. Our taste alone can no longer be an adequate guide in today's environment of sprayed, processed, commercialized, and chemicalized foods. Dependable nutritional information is needed if we are to get the best performance from our bodies — and enable them to last as long as possible.

Many people today are restricting their use of meat because they wish to live in greater harmony with their environment or to avoid saturated fats. The Food Table has information on non-meat sources of protein that are much easier on the budget than meat — and most likely easier on your arteries, too.

One unique feature of the book is the Vitamin-Mineral Index. So far as I know, this is an original scientific yardstick that gives you an indication of the vitamin and mineral contribution that a food makes in your diet. For example, white sugar, which has no vitamins or minerals, has a zero Vitamin-Mineral Index. The V-M Index of whole milk is 8. Skim milk, which has the fat removed, has a V-M Index of 14 because you get more vitamins and minerals *per calorie* than with the whole milk. Any food that is low on calories and high on vitamins and minerals will have a high Vitamin-Mineral Index. For example, raw cabbage has a V-M Index of 58. This Index can be particularly helpful to individuals who wish to keep their weight down and at the same time increase their nutrition! If you go through the Food Table beginning on page 217 and emphasize those foods in your diet which have a V-M Index of 25 or above, *you can instantly double or triple the vitamins and minerals in your diet.*

Loving Your Body is the result of a scientific study of the nutritional needs of the human body. I completed work on this book almost seven years before the chain of circumstances that led me to the formulation of the Living Love "Science of Happiness." I now recognize that *Loving Your Body* is part of a trilogy that summarizes my work on myself — in terms of body, mind, and spirit . . . The previous book, *How to Develop Your Thinking Ability,* represents a summary of the way I developed my mind to make it a useful helper to me. The *Handbook to Higher Consciousness* enables me to share with other people the liberating techniques that let me free my spirit from the many motivational chains I had unknowingly forged to keep it a prisoner.

Our bodies may most fruitfully be regarded as temples that house our consciousness and make possible its continuation. In our essence, we are not our bodies — any more than we are our rational minds, our emotions, our programming, or our egos. That essence of a human being which sets us apart from animals is our capacity to be *consciously aware of the consequences of the role in the drama that we are playing in our everyday life activities.*

A healthy, energetic body is a help in assisting us to spring free from the ego-backed illusions that keep us from living a perceptive, wise, conscious, loving, peaceful, happy, and fulfilling life. One's growth toward higher consciousness depends on liberating oneself from being compulsively gripped by the negative, alienating emotions that are triggered by one's security, sensation, and power programming. One's world becomes a warm, friendly place in which to live when our experience of the here and now in our lives is generated by the beautiful motivations associated with accepting and loving everyone unconditionally — including oneself.

Ken Keyes, Jr.
Berkeley, California
August, 1974.

Chapter 1

ON MICE AND MEN

Modern nutrition is a gold mine that can help you add more life to your years—and more years to your life. These pages have been written to show you how to use the latest findings of nutritional science to help you:

1. Maintain a full-of-life energy level.
2. Raise your defenses to infection and disease.
3. Lengthen your period of sexual virility.
4. Add many *vigorous* years to your life.

This book, which is hot off the scientific griddle, gives you four pioneering features not available in other books on nutrition:

1. It is the only book that offers *a simple way* to analyze the nutrients in your daily diet. You will be able to see how well or how poorly you are now nourishing yourself—and the loved ones in your family.

2. In Chapter 20 you will find a Nutrition Test that will enable you to measure how well you are doing nutritionally at the present time. When you know your Nutrition Score, you can compare it with others in your family. The test can also show you how rapidly you are improving your diet.

3. This book explains how to use the Vitamin-Mineral Index, which can help you choose foods high in vitamins and minerals. This scientific rating of the vitamin-mineral content of foods is *completely new*.

4. You will also find the most *useful* Food Table available today. It is one of the first Food Tables to show the amount of dangerous saturated fat in each food. You can reduce your chances of a coronary heart attack by applying the information on saturated and unsaturated fats found in Chapter 7.

You will discover in the chapter on protein a way to keep your energy at a high level throughout the entire day. Other chapters will show you how you can benefit from the extensive knowledge of vitamins and minerals that science has made available. Have you tried to lose weight without success? The chapter on weight control debunks a lot of current nonsense and explains in easy-to-follow terms a method that has proven effective for lifetime weight control. And just so you won't worry about placing added strain on an already overloaded budget, the last chapter explains how you can actually reduce the amount of money you spend for foods and at the same time greatly increase the nutritional value of your meals!

SEVENTY GENERATIONS OF RATS

"From the standpoint of health," says Hazel K. Stiebeling of the U.S. Department of Agriculture, "better diets could mean smaller outlays for illness, less loss of working time, greater physical efficiency, and longer, more productive life." [1] To begin our exploration of

1. J. P. Cavin, Hazel K. Stiebeling, and Marius Farioletti, "Agricultural Surpluses and Nutritional Deficits," from *Farmers in a Changing World, The Yearbook of Agriculture 1940*, p. 334. (Washington, D.C.: U.S. Government Printing Office, 1940.)

this fascinating subject of modern nutrition, let's look into the laboratory of the late Dr. Henry C. Sherman, who was associated with Columbia University for sixty years. In 1920, Dr. Sherman and his co-workers began a farsighted experiment. They took a group of bright-eyed white rats and fed them a diet of one-sixth whole milk powder, five-sixths ground whole wheat, plus table salt and water. Dr. Sherman called this "Diet A," and the rats were invited to eat all they wanted. About thirty years later, Dr. Sherman had raised over seventy generations on Diet A, and they were still going strong! He considered this an *adequate* diet because the rats thrived and reproduced well.

But who is going to be satisfied with something simply adequate? Certainly not Dr. Sherman. Through his experiments with animals, he felt that men deserve something better. We should have *optimal nutrition*. And optimal nutrition means *the very best possible*.

Using Diet A as a yardstick against which he could measure improvements, Dr. Sherman decided to alter the proportions of milk and wheat. The new Sherman "Diet B" contained one-third dried whole milk, two-thirds ground whole wheat, plus table salt and water. This gave the rats twice as much milk, and since milk is an excellent source of calcium, vitamin A, and vitamin B_2, the amounts of these vital nutrients were increased. Dr. Sherman found that this simple change in the rats' diet produced surprising gains in health and vitality. There was a longer period of sexual performance. Rats on Diet B raised 120 per cent more young ones, and there was a decrease in the percentage of females who failed to bear and raise young. Old age was deferred for the mother rats, as evidenced by a 73 per cent longer reproductive life. But perhaps the most thrilling part of Diet B was the effect it had on the life span of the rats. The girl rats increased their longevity by 10.9 per cent! The boy rats increased their average life span by 11.2 per cent! [2]

STAY YOUNGER LONGER

Dr. Sherman's famous experiment challenged the long-accepted idea that our life span is determined only by heredity. "There had been previous studies of longevity, made by very different methods which enabled investigators to correlate longevity with heredity and with nothing else," Dr. Sherman commented in his scientific style. "Under those conditions it came to be assumed and was taught, far too dogmatically, that 'we cannot add years to our lives though we can add life to our years' and that 'there are many ways in which we can shorten our lives but the only way to lengthen them is by the selection of a longer-lived ancestry.'

"Such teaching," said Dr. Sherman, "can now be seen to be misleading because it states only a part of the truth as if it were the whole; and it is not true to the spirit of science because it is fatalistic and tends to close the mind. The new evidence of full-life research now shows that *nutrition as well as heredity* is a major factor in determining the length of life. It is now clearly incorrect to believe that the length of our lives will be determined exclusively by our heredity. Heredity will have its influence, but food habits will have their influence as well. We cannot select our ancestors, but can select our foods. We can and should *both* add life to our years *and* add years to our lives." [3]

After hearing about the rats on Diet B, one attractive woman wrote me, "I hate to think of all those

2. Henry C. Sherman, *The Nutritional Improvement of Life*, pp. 71–75. (New York: Columbia University Press, 1950.)
3. *Ibid.*, p. 5.

rats on Diet B living longer, bearing more ratlets, and getting all those vitamins that could be put to a better use by another brand of animal. . . . Also, stop making us females, whether rodent or human, bear longer. You'll fix it so a woman is never safe!" Of course, added fertility and virility are only a part of the added life for added years that improved nutrition may bring you.

ADEQUATE *VS.* OPTIMAL NUTRITION

Dr. Sherman's experiments led him to the conclusion that ". . . certain nutrients consumed in higher than hitherto usual amounts may increase the normal adult life expectation by about a decade—and this not added to old age but inserted at the apex of the prime of life." [4] In spite of the great improvements in vitality and longevity given by Diet B, Dr. Sherman did not regard it as *optimal*—that is, so good that it could not be improved.

People who worked with Winston Churchill found he was "easily satisfied with the best—no less." This, too, should be our goal in nutrition. Dr. E. V. McCollum of Johns Hopkins University has suggested that we cease thinking of nutrition only in terms of avoiding deficiency. He pointed out that nutrition has not only a preventative aspect, but a positive health-building aspect as well. Dr. McCollum emphasized the difference between merely *adequate* nutrition and *optimal* nutrition.[5] To him an optimal diet has the following characteristics:

1. Promotes good growth.
2. Permits the highest fertility in the female and the highest virility in the male.

4. *Ibid.*, p. 164.
5. *Ibid.*, pp. 67–70.

3. Gives the highest level of success in rearing healthy youngsters.
4. Preserves youth and delays senility.
5. Extends the life span to the limit.

If you are too young to feel as old as you feel, optimal nutrition should be your goal. The *Journal of the American Medical Association* has remarked editorially that "there is a real difference as measured in terms of growth, development and general health record betwen optimum and just adequate nutrition; and that every practical effort should be made to apply this knowledge in the interests of human welfare." [6] Life jumps into a new dimension when you begin to enjoy the many benefits of optimal nutrition. This book will show you step-by-step how to work toward this exciting goal.

Chapter 2

IF YOU'RE THICK AND TIRED OF IT

Many years ago (before I became interested in nutrition), I had polio and have been in a wheel chair ever since. Somehow my appetite never got the word, and I like to eat as though I were digging ditches all day. I am tempted not only by gourmet foods, but by almost all foods. Year after year I added weight, despite what seemed to be intelligent attempts to control it. I cut out butter, stayed away from bread, trimmed the fat off meat, avoided sweets, and still the pounds piled on.

My break-even point on calories is somewhere around 1,250 per day—about one-half of the normal amount. For most people this is a rigorous reducing diet, yet for me it is a level I must live with. But if I need only 1,250 calories daily, how in the world do I go about losing weight? For a while it seemed to me that the only answer would be simply to get into a straitjacket and stay there for the number of months required to reduce. Every time I tried cutting down on calories, my energy would drag bottom. This interfered with my work; it interfered with everything. Soon the calories began flowing again and I had one more chunk of evidence to prove the hopelessness of keeping my weight down. I was trapped in my own fat.

Matters stayed like this for years, with the pounds adding up all the time. Then I became interested in nutrition. I was attracted primarily by the added energy and zest for living, the higher degree of health, and promise of greater longevity. I still regarded the control of my weight as an all but impossible task. As my interest in nutrition expanded into the study of optimal nutrition, I began to learn many helpful things.

I found that on a diet of 1,250 calories I could pack in more protein than most people get from 2,000 to 3,000 calories. I learned the importance of using certain foods that are heavily loaded with vitamins and minerals. I discovered that by *increasing my protein, vitamins, and minerals while holding down on calories,* I was able gradually to control my weight—and at the same time maintain a high level of energy that permitted me to carry on a busy life. If you have the problem of excess pounds, I'd like to share with you the things I have learned.

THE PRICE OF OBESITY

Up until the twentieth century, a generous amount of fat on your body was considered a sign of affluence, beauty, and health. Today, the only premium attached to excess pounds is in life insurance policies. And this is a penalty, rather than a tribute. When a life insurance company writes your policy, they base the premium on your expected life span. If you die sooner, they lose money. If you live longer, they make money on you.

The countless hours that the life insurance statisticians have devoted to the problem of obesity can be summed up briefly: "The longer the belt line, the shorter the life line." They find that even if you are only 10 per cent overweight, you are in a group that has a *mortality or death rate one-third higher than if you are within the desirable weight range.* To see how you're doing, check the table that follows. For men 20 per cent overweight, the excess mortality is about one-half. This means that they have a 50 per cent greater chance of dying any given year as compared with those with desirable weights. Women also tend to have shorter life spans when they have bulgy silhouettes, but the toll they pay for this extra poundage is not as heavy as for men. People who run 5 to 10 per cent *underweight* have a slightly increased life expectancy. Edward A. Lew, Actuary and Statistician of the Metropolitan Life Insurance Company, suggests that for greatest longevity you keep your weight down to about what you weighed in your early twenties.[1]

REDUCING PAYS OFF

What about those who have been fat for many years, but who reduce and keep their weight down? Will they be rewarded with added years? Fortunately, this pays off both in lower life insurance premiums and in greater longevity. Men who averaged as much as 35 per cent overweight at the time they were insured, achieved an almost normal life expectancy upon reducing, and their insurance premiums were correspondingly reduced.

If you overload a two-ton truck day after day, you can't expect it to give years of good service. The same thing applies to our bodies. The human skeleton is not well adapted to carrying around an extra load of fat. Flat feet and arthritis of the knees, hips, and spine are common in corpulent people. Blood circulation may be

1. Edward A. Lew, "New Data on Underweight and Overweight Persons," *Journal of The American Dietetic Association,* Vol. 38, p. 324, 1961.

DESIRABLE WEIGHTS

Ages 25 and Over

Height (without shoes)	Weight Without Clothing		
	Small frame	Medium frame	Large frame
MEN			
	pounds	*pounds*	*pounds*
5 ft. 1 in.	104-112	110-121	118-133
5 ft. 2 in.	107-115	113-125	121-136
5 ft. 3 in.	110-118	116-128	124-140
5 ft. 4 in.	113-121	119-131	127-144
5 ft. 5 in.	116-125	122-135	130-148
5 ft. 6 in.	120-129	126-139	134-153
5 ft. 7 in.	124-133	130-144	139-158
5 ft. 8 in.	128-137	134-148	143-162
5 ft. 9 in.	132-142	138-152	147-166
5 ft. 10 in.	136-146	142-157	151-171
5 ft. 11 in.	140-150	146-162	156-176
6 ft.	144-154	150-167	160-181
6 ft. 1 in.	148-159	154-172	165-186
6 ft. 2 in.	152-163	159-177	170-191
6 ft. 3 in.	156-167	164-182	174-196
WOMEN			
4 ft. 8 in.	87- 93	91-102	99-114
4 ft. 9 in.	89- 96	93-105	101-117
4 ft. 10 in.	91- 99	96-108	104-120
4 ft. 11 in.	94-102	99-111	107-123
5 ft.	97-105	102-114	110-126
5 ft. 1 in.	100-108	105-117	113-129
5 ft. 2 in.	103-111	108-121	116-133
5 ft. 3 in.	106-114	111-125	120-137
5 ft. 4 in.	109-118	115-130	124-141
5 ft. 5 in.	113-122	119-134	128-145
5 ft. 6 in.	117-126	123-138	132-149
5 ft. 7 in.	121-130	127-142	136-153
5 ft. 8 in.	125-135	131-146	140-158
5 ft. 9 in.	129-139	135-150	144-163
5 ft. 10 in.	133-143	139-154	148-168

For weights with ordinary indoor clothing, add 5 pounds for women and 8 pounds for men to the above figures.

Adapted from New Weight Standards for Men and Women, published by the Metropolitan Life Insurance Company, 1959.

poor with resulting hernias and varicose veins. Extra fat around your diaphragm may keep you from breathing freely, and this leaves the way open to coughs and bronchitis. Increased chances of gout and diabetes are additional risks run by those with swollen figures. When obese people require surgery, the doctors sweat it out with them, for they are much greater risks than folks of normal weight. "Obesity," says Dr. Stanley Davidson, ". . . gives rise to more ill-health than all the vitamin deficiencies put together." [2]

The physical penalties paid by those who are overloaded with extra pounds are perhaps light compared with the mental pains they endure. The unattractiveness of the stout figure leads to embarrassment and a sensitivity to ridicule that hurts deeply. Most corpulent people would dearly love to shed these hated pounds. They have tried time and time again, only to meet with failure. Sometimes they succeed in removing a few layers of fat, but within six months to a year these unwanted pounds return. No person of normal weight can possibly appreciate the hellish torments of someone trying to lose twenty-five or fifty pounds. Fortunately the road toward optimal nutrition can help you if you want to reduce your weight—whether your problem is ten pounds or a hundred pounds.

FRAUDULENT DIETS

It is small wonder that so many people have become discouraged about reducing. Few subjects have more hogwash written about them. You have seen diets that promised a weight loss of five pounds in two days. The loss of this much *fat* through diet in a 48-

2. Stanley Davidson, A. P. Meiklejohn, and R. Passmore, *Human Nutrition and Dietetics,* p. 386. (Baltimore: The Williams and Wilkins Co., 1959.)

hour period is impossible. Here's why. Every pound
of fat you have stored in your body represents about
3,500 stored calories.[3] Let us suppose that your body
requires 2,300 calories per day. This means that if you
ate nothing whatsoever you still would not burn up
a pound of fat in a day!

You can thus see how ridiculous it is to claim that
a reducing diet will help you take off five pounds of
fat in two days. Five pounds of fat at 3,500 calories
per pound amounts to 17,500 calories. A person who
requires 2,300 calories per day would not lose five
pounds of *fat* even if he ate nothing for a whole week!

The first step in controlling your weight is to
understand the problem correctly. Think of each pound
of fat tucked away in those bulges as representing 3,500
stored calories. Whenever you eat 3,500 calories more
than you need to meet your energy requirements, you
have deposited another pound in your fat bank. Whenever you burn up 3,500 calories more than you have
eaten, you are withdrawing a pound of fat from your
bank. Keep up the withdrawals and you'll soon be
able to take in your belt or slip into those chic torea-
dor pants again.

I find it helpful to think of losing *ounces* of fat.
There are 16 ounces in a pound. Since a pound represents about 3,500 stored calories, an ounce of fat
is equal to about 220 calories. Thus, if I overeat by 220
calories, I gain an ounce. If I'm 220 calories under my
needs for the day, I lose an ounce. If I'm shy 440 calories, I lose 2 ounces. A loss of 2 ounces a day adds up
to 14 ounces a week. Over a period of a month I have,
presto! lost about four pounds. Watch the ounces and
the pounds take care of themselves.

3. Michael G. Wohl, "Obesity," from Michael G. Wohl and
Robert S. Goodhart, eds., *Modern Nutrition in Health and Disease*,
p. 865. (Philadelphia: Lea and Febiger, 1960.)

UNREALISTIC IDEAS

People who are overweight usually have a lot of reasons why they are as they are. Many of these folks can point to a long line of fat ancestors. Thus they develop a feeling that it's probably inherited, and therefore not their fault. It should always be remembered that while body build is inherited, obesity is not. "A more realistic explanation," said Dr. L. H. Newburgh, "is the continuation of the familial tradition of the groaning board and the savory dish." [4] Some people blame the tension of modern life for weighing one hundred and plenty. Food helps them allay anxiety, worry, and frustration. "Food," said Dr. Michael Wohl, "is their liquor." [5]

Many folks who are overweight have a "reason" that leaves them blameless—"My doctor says it's my glands." They are probably wrong. But regardless of whatever factors may play a part, there is only one basic cause for being overweight: THEY ARE EATING MORE CALORIES THAN THEY ARE BURNING UP. Fat does not come out of the air. Its origin is the dinner plate or cocktail glass—it's as simple as that.

There are only two basic solutions to this problem:
1. Hold down your calories and/or
2. Burn up more calories.

WASTED EFFORTS

Sometimes it seems that folks are determined to try everything except the right thing. Stout folks have

4. L. H. Newburgh, "Obesity," from Norman Jolliffe, F. F. Tisdall, and Paul R. Cannon, eds., *Clinical Nutrition*, p. 720. (New York: Hoeber Medical Division, Harper & Row, Publishers, Inc., 1950.)
5. Wohl, *op. cit.*, p. 860.

tried massage, hot baths, cold baths, hot showers, cold showers, Turkish baths, Scotch douches, Russian baths, steam baths, and electric light cabinets. When you sit there sweating away in a hot bath, you can lose as much as two pounds of water per hour—and nary a speck of fat.[6]

Men put a great deal of emphasis on reducing their waistlines and women seem chiefly concerned about reducing their hips. Both sexes jointly work on the "double chin." Billions have been spent for pills and drugs, slenderizing creams, lotions, and bath powders, bulk fillers, reducing belts, chin straps, rollers, and massaging devices. The loss in dollars has been great; the loss in pounds negligible.

We have been subjected to the all-fruit diet, the green vegetable diet, the potato diet, the pineapple and lamb chop diet, the royal tomato and hard-boiled egg diet, and the bread and butter diet. One especially interesting reducing diet even included martinis; this, I understand, was given a thorough test by many people.

Some companies are now offering food made from calorieless cellulose. But Dr. Herbert Pollack of the American Diabetes Association says, "The whole point ought to be to re-educate people's eating habits—to eat two pancakes instead of six—rather than to rely on what may prove to be another fad and perhaps even a digestive-tract irritant."

A new wrinkle is the 900-calorie liquid formula diets. They have the advantage of saving you from counting calories or facing the tempting sight of food. However, the Council on Foods and Nutrition of the A.M.A. does not endorse these diets. They caution, "One of the most important goals in any long-term

6. Frank H. Krusen, "Physical Medicine and Obesity," *Journal of the American Medical Association*, Vol. 151, pp. 296-297, 1953.

weight control program is that of educating the patient in good and bad dietary habits. This type of education is best achieved by building the therapeutic diet around ordinary foods." [7]

The method of reducing described in this chapter can help you achieve lifetime control of your weight and avoid what Dr. Jean Mayer of Harvard described as "the rhythm method of girth control." Fat-thin-fat-again tends to build up cholesterol in your arteries and encourage the formation of gallstones, in addition to playing havoc with your wardrobe. One plump person I know goes through this cycle every year. She arranges her closet in sections: size 14, 16, 18, and 20!

OPTIMAL WEIGHT REDUCTION

When a doctor advised his bulging patient that the best thing for her health was to cut down on calories, she replied, "Frankly, I don't deserve the best. What's the next best?" Unfortunately there is no "next best" road to slimming. It all gets back to a matter of bookkeeping. If you're shy 220 calories for the day, you will lose an ounce of weight. If you eat 220 more than you need, you will gain an ounce of weight. There is no short cut, no magic way out, and no court of appeal from this tough reality.

The first step in optimal weight reduction is to find out how many calories you need each day *to maintain the weight you prefer to have.* To do this, simply multiply your desired weight in pounds by 15 if you are moderately active. For example, if you want to weigh 150 pounds, your diet should contain no more than 2,250 calories each day to maintain your present

7. *Journal of the American Medical Association,* Vol. 176, p. 439, 1961.

weight (150 pounds $\times$ 15 = 2,250 calories). You will recall that there are approximately 3,500 calories stored in each pound of fat. Thus, if you want to lose one pound a week, you must undereat by 500 calories each day.

Here, step by step, is a way to approach optimal weight reduction:

1. Multiply your present weight by 15 to get the number of calories you need each day to maintain your present weight.

2. Subtract 500 calories from this figure. This will give you a deficit of 3,500 calories a week which will enable you to lose about a pound a week. This is your daily calorie budget while reducing.*

3. Using the Food Table that begins on Page 217, plan a diet that stays within this calorie budget.

4. Make sure that your reducing diet meets the nutritional standards of this book. You can boost your protein intake with seafoods, cottage cheese, skim milk, and other foods high in protein but low in calories. Chapter 9 explains the Vitamin-Mineral Index—a new, simple guide that indicates the concentration of vitamins and minerals in each food. To keep your energy at the highest possible level, use vegetables and fruits that have Vitamin-Mineral Indexes higher than 25. This helpful guide appears in the next to the last column of the Food Table in the back of this book.

The above four steps are the heart of the most effective method known for simultaneously increasing your energy and decreasing your weight. It will assure you a diet that is rich in all nutrients except calories. It

---

* Underweight people who wish to gain should *add* 500 calories per day to their maintenance level. Several extra tablespoons of vegetable oil each day can add many calories with little filling bulk.

WILL HELP YOU CUT DOWN ON CALORIES BUT NOT ON
FOOD.

DON'T TRY TO REDUCE TOO FAST

People get into trouble when they try to take
off weight too rapidly. It deprives them of energy
needed to meet the tempo of modern living. Except for
those with an iron will or those who had the pants
scared off them by their doctor, they will soon "cheat"
on a severe diet. Even if your will power can stand
the strain of a severe reducing diet, your body may
not. It throws an added burden on your heart and other
organs. Your skin becomes wrinkled after a rapid loss
of fat and you'll look haggard. And what's worse—
your disposition will be awful.

It is dangerous to try a heroic fast to get your
weight down in a hurry. The rapid breakdown of fat
stored in your body without some carbohydrate in your
diet will have toxic effects. Barbara Hutton, the Wool-
worth heiress, whose slender figure set fashion styles,
found that she had gained ten unwanted pounds. She
went on a coffee diet, drinking sixteen cups of strong
black coffee each day with vitamin pills "to make sure
I stay healthy." The result was a serious intestinal
obstruction, a mad dash for the hospital, and an emergency operation.

A weight loss of one pound per week may be an
optimal rate for reducing. The fatter you are, the more
important it may be to reduce slowly.

ON YOUR WAY TOWARD A SLIMMER FIGURE

While you are rearranging your body contours,
make sure that you continue to work toward optimal
nutrition. Proper amounts of protein, fat, vitamins, and

minerals are more vital than ever. You need the best possible nutrition to meet this stress. You may be surprised that I am not advising you to cut down on fats. As explained in Chapter 6, your body needs fat to carry vitamins and minerals into your blood stream. Essential linoleic fat has many jobs to do while you are taking off these pounds. Don't compromise on any part of your program of optimal nutrition—except on calories.

Too many square meals may make too many round figures. I have found that I can control my weight best when I eat about eight small snacks instead of the usual three meals a day. Dr. Clarence Cohn has shown that animals eating their food *in meals* tended to gain more fat than animals that *"nibble"* throughout the day.[8] He found many health benefits including lower cholesterol among animals that nibble occasionally instead of eating meals. In my personal program of weight control, I find that eating small amounts of nutritious food every hour or two throughout the day helps me avoid the hunger that is such a strong invitation to overeating. I have also found that I enjoy a higher level of intestinal health when I go in for "nibbling" instead of "meal eating."

A nutritionist once said that the only exercise needed for weight control is the exercise of intelligence. It is often pointed out that you have to walk about thirty-five miles to take off a pound of fat. It is also correct that a round of golf or game of tennis on the weekend won't make a great deal of difference in your weight. Nevertheless I think we should still say a kind word for exercise. There is no doubt that our bodies can probably benefit from far more muscular activity than our modern push-button lives give us. There is a

8. Clarence Cohn and Dorothy Joseph, "Effects on Metabolism Produced by the Rate of Ingestion of the Diet," *American Journal of Clinical Nutrition*, Vol. 8, pp. 682-690, 1960.

real value in developing a daily pattern of exercise that fits in with your way of life. Suppose, for example, you take a half-hour stroll each evening after dinner. Walking outdoors uses calories about four times faster than watching television. A thirty-minute walk after dinner may result in removing several pounds of fat per year, and it may have many other benefits besides.

Don't expect immediate results when you begin your program of weight control. Scientists have found that sometimes a person will lose fat for as long as two weeks without losing *a pound of weight!* When fat is lost, it may be replaced by water, and your scales won't tell you the full story. A pint of water held in your body adds one pound to your weight. Women often gain two to three pounds of water during menstruation. They can be losing fat and gaining weight at the same time! Your normal weight will vary by a pound or so each day due to the seesawing of food intake, water intake, and elimination. This may be disheartening if the scales are watched too closely. It is best to weigh yourself once every week or two and to stay on your program day in and day out regardless of what your scales tell you.

You'll be fooling yourself if you cut out salt when reducing. Salt restriction will cause your body to lose pounds of water, but not pounds of fat. It may temporarily improve your morale to quickly lose several "phony" pounds—but how will you feel when you regain these pounds of water?

Often it will take four to six weeks for you to train your appetite to adjust to your program of optimal reducing. Patience is required. Some people find it helpful to eat slowly and get more enjoyment from smaller quantities. Raw vegetables, such as carrots and celery, are very filling. It's smart to plan ahead so that you will have a graceful way to turn down offers of cocktails, desserts, or extra foods when in company.

The big thing to remember in your reducing diet (as well as in your normal program of optimal nutrition) is to *make every calorie count*. Stay away from the "emptier" calories. Try to make up for a lack of calories by an increase in your protein, vitamins, and minerals. Experiment on paper with your Nutrition Analysis Form (explained in Chapter 19) to see how much of these other nutrients you can get in your daily diet without fracturing your calorie budget.

If you follow this program of optimal reducing, you will find the unwanted pounds will melt away gradually and safely, probably never to return. Such a program is the opposite of a crash diet. When you have achieved that beautiful weight you want, you will have a pattern of nutrition that will give you firm control of your weight. It has been estimated that 90 per cent of the people who lose a large amount of weight will regain it within six months to a year. With your new knowledge of nutrition, you won't have to go through *that* again.

Chapter 3

SUSTAINING ENERGY WITH PROTEIN

In 1858 a Dutch physician, Gerrit Jan Mulder, announced that all living plants and animals are made from a certain substance without which life is impossible. He named it "protein" from a Greek word that means "first place."

When you look at yourself in a mirror you see a superb package of protein. Your skin, your hair, and your nails—even the basic framework of your teeth and bones—are protein. Body tissues cannot be built without protein. The rest of your body, which you cannot see—heart, arteries, kidneys, lungs, brain, and intestinal organs, and even genes that blueprint your heredity—is made of protein, too.

When you increased your body cells from one to about twenty-six trillion during your first twenty years, you used protein to build every one of them. In a growing infant up to one-third of the protein in his milk may be used for building new tissues. The wear and tear department of your body must replace millions of cells daily. Your twenty-five billion red blood cells, for example, have an average life of only 120 days.

Fortunately, our bodies can reprocess some of this worn out protein.

Injury or loss of blood will increase your need for protein. This basic nutrient is a part of most of your vital body fluids. Your red and white blood cells, the hormones that chemically regulate your body processes, and the enzymes that spark the incredibly complex chemical reactions within your body are all proteins. This nutrient plays an essential part in maintaining the proper water balance of your body. If it is inadequate, extra water may be drawn into your tissues and swelling can occur. Some people who think they are overweight are mainly waterlogged due to poor nutrition.

Protein is a versatile nutrient. Depending on your needs, it can have either an acid or an alkaline effect on your blood. Many years ago there was much ado over getting a proper proportion of acid and alkaline foods in the diet. Because of the versatility of protein and your body's other ingenious ways of regulating your acid-alkaline balance, you can forget about this in your quest for optimal nutrition.

Enzymes that digest your food require protein. Unless you have an adequate supply of digestive juices, many of the nutritive values of the food you eat will go down the drain. The complex hormones that control the many delicate adjustments needed to keep your body functioning are made from protein. These include thyroxine made by the thyroid gland; insulin produced by the pancreas; adrenalin from the adrenal glands. Proteins also are vital to the production of antibodies that help ward off infection, and phagocytes that eat up invading bacteria.

A mild protein deficiency can undermine health. Dr. E. V. McCollum found that mice raised on a good diet except for protein maintained health for a while, but eventually they showed lower fertility, evidences of disease, and early senility.[1]

They say that you're getting old when you start throwing kisses instead of delivering them. Adequate protein may slow down the rate of aging. It has been found that young men on a diet restricted in protein were definitely depressed in sex drive even when it produced no other observable effect! [2] Dr. L. E. Holt found that a protein deficiency resulted in a decrease in sperm formation and mobility of sperm in men.[3]

It has been found that too little protein produces grouchiness, lack of appetite, and tiredness, which are relieved when the protein intake becomes adequate. In severe protein deficiency, your skin loses its soft elastic character and looks dry and scaly. It breaks down easily and slight wounds are slow to heal and become infected quickly.

If you omit protein from your diet, your body will steal it from your less essential tissues to keep you alive. Scientific experiments with protein-starved rats showed that 40 per cent of the protein in the liver could be requisitioned in an emergency to preserve life. They also used up 5 per cent of the protein in their brains, 8 per cent was taken from the muscles and skin, and 30 per cent from the digestive tract.[4] Dr. G. Lusk has estimated that a protein-starved man may manage to

1. E. V. McCollum, N. Simmonds, and H. T. Parsons, "Supplementary Protein Values in Foods; Supplementary Dietary Relations between Proteins of Cereal Grains and Potato," *Journal of Biological Chemistry*, Vol. 47, p. 175, 1921.

2. James S. McLester and William J. Darby, *Nutrition and Diet in Health and Disease*, 6th ed., p. 56. (Philadelphia: W. B. Saunders Company, 1952.)

3. L. E. Holt, Jr. and A. A. Albanese, "Observations on Amino Acid Deficiencies in Man," *Transactions of the Association of American Physicians*, Vol. 58, p. 143, 1944.

4. T. Addis, L. J. Poo, and W. Lew, *Journal of Biological Chemistry*, Vol. 116, p. 343, 1936.

live about a year by robbing his own tissues if carbo-hydrates are adequately supplied.

Building a high level of health without protein is like trying to sew without thread. It just can't be done. Your body, however, has a remarkable ability to adjust itself and, if necessary, can get along on two-thirds of the protein contained in the recommended allowances of the National Research Council.

HOW PROTEIN HELPS SUSTAIN YOUR ENERGY

Your vim and vigor depend on the level of sugar in your blood stream. When your blood circulates an adequate supply of sugar to all of the cells of your body, life can be beautiful. When your blood-sugar level is low, you feel tired and edgy. If it is low enough, you may even get nauseated or faint. Most people think of soft drinks and candy bars as a way to quick energy. The trouble is, it's too quick. Sugar is quickly absorbed and quickly gone. Protein, however, is processed slowly by your digestive system. When eaten in adequate quantities *it will promote a sustained energy level for hours.*

The usual breakfast of cereal, toast, jelly, and coffee only contains about 10 per cent of your protein allowance for the day. Such a high carbohydrate break-fast has quickly digested starches and sugars that prob-ably send your blood sugar sky-rocketing an hour after eating. It may be quick energy, but it doesn't last long. When the blood-sugar level gets too high, the pancreas squirts a shot of insulin into the blood to pull it down. If the blood-sugar level rises too much too fast, insulin may be oversupplied. About an hour and a half after eating, this excess insulin can leave you with a lower blood-sugar level than when you got up. This midmorn-ing letdown often leads to a candy bar, soft drink, or pastry—all of which are high in sugar and calories and low or missing in protein. Again, your blood sugar skyrockets and is quickly knocked down by insulin so that you end up at lunchtime ready to ride the same seesaw again.

To help you achieve and sustain a high energy level, you need a high protein breakfast with a reasonable amount of carbohydrate. Dr. George Thorn at Harvard University tested three types of breakfast—one high in carbohydrate, one high in fat, and the third high in protein.[5] The high carbohydrate meal contained orange juice, corn flakes, sugar, bread, butter, jelly, and milk. An hour after this starchy and sugary breakfast, the blood sugar jumped too high, and one hour later it nosedived. Then it started to climb slowly but even three hours afterward it had only returned to the prebreakfast level. Hunger and weakness developed between the second and third hour after breakfast, setting up a craving for a between-meal snack.

When the high fat breakfast of heavy cream and corn flakes was eaten, Dr. Thorn found that the blood-sugar level gradually fell for five hours. Hunger was felt but the symptoms were not as severe as with the high carbohydrate breakfast.

When the high protein breakfast consisting of skim milk, lean beef, and cottage cheese was eaten, a normal blood-sugar level was maintained for six hours afterward! This energy breakfast contained about three-quarters of the daily protein allowance. *"A definite sense of well-being" was reported during this entire six-hour period.*

Investigators at Iowa State University found that

5. G. W. Thorn, J. T. Quimby, and M. Clinton, Jr., "A Comparison of the Metabolic Effects of Isocaloric Meals of Varying Composition, with Special Reference to the Prevention of Postprandial Hypoglycemic Symptoms," *Annals of Internal Medicine*, Vol. 18, p. 913, 1943.

when you get about a third of your daily allowance of protein for breakfast, your blood sugar will remain at an energy-sustaining level for about three and one-half hours. They also confirmed that a high protein breakfast raises the blood-sugar level more slowly and sustains it for a longer time. The breakfast filled with starches and sugars led to a midmorning slump and a craving for a between-meal snack.

They made many tests and found that work efficiency was lowered when breakfast was omitted or when coffee alone was taken.[6] When you eat a low protein breakfast, you not only cheat yourself, but you also cheat your boss. It does not matter what type of protein you eat. Either animal or vegetable protein does the trick if the amount equals at least one-third of your daily protein allowance.[7]

The idea of an energy-sustaining breakfast is not new. During the last century in this country, breakfast frequently consisted of eggs, meat, porridge, hot breads, coffee cake, fruit pies, pickles, and broiled fish or fowl. In 1958 at the National Food Conference in Washington, D.C., Vice President Nixon, in his keynote address, put the spotlight on our poor breakfast habits: ". . . only 12 per cent of the people of the United States eat what we would call a good breakfast. About 62 per cent eat what is termed a fair breakfast but not an adequate one, and 26 per cent eat one which is not adequate at all, or a poor breakfast."

How many people do you know that have little or no breakfast, a snack for lunch, and then try to make up for this bodily insult by a hearty supper? Such

6. W. W. Tuttle, K. Daum, L. Myers, and C. Martin, *Journal of the American Dietetic Association*, Vol. 26, p. 332, 1950.
7. V. E. Addison, W. W. Tuttle, K. Daum, and R. Larsen, "Effect of Amount and Type of Protein in Breakfasts on Blood Sugar Levels," *Journal of the American Dietetic Association*, Vol. 29, p. 674, 1953.

a pattern provides us with low blood-sugar levels during the busy day but with high levels when we should be ready for sleep. Any engineer of a ship who let the steam pressure fall when the ship headed out of port, but who kept a full head of steam whenever it got to the dock would be fired.

A LION-SIZED BREAKFAST

To maintain a desirable weight and remain at maximum efficiency, try eating like a lion for breakfast, like a squirrel for lunch, and like a bird for supper. If you eat a large supper and go to sleep a few hours later, all through the night you are building fat cells like mad. You wake up a little closer to a bay window and a triple chin.

Some people think that by skipping breakfast they can keep their weight down. Actually it's just the opposite. By having a high protein breakfast, you will tend to *increase your activity and burn up calories faster*. You will sit more erectly and move more energetically.

When a fat person was asked by a dietician to write down her typical meal pattern, she wrote: "Breakfast—coffee. Lunch—almost anything. Supper—the same." Her lack of protein for breakfast could have been partly responsible for the excess blubber. An adequate breakfast might have prevented overeating later in the day.

Many people report that their craving for sweets is reduced when they use a high protein breakfast. Sometimes the excessive use of cigarettes, coffee, and alcohol may be due to a low blood-sugar level. These stimulants may not be needed when you eat a high protein breakfast to sustain energy and vitality. How's your disposition lately? No one can be at his best when his blood sugar is dragging bottom throughout a busy day.

Nationwide surveys have shown that only one out of every five children goes to school with an adequate breakfast. A midmorning slump in blood-sugar level may be depriving your children of the energy they need to do good work at school. Research has shown that more interest in learning and better report cards may result when the youngsters go to school well fortified with protein.[8]

Some of the beneficial results of optimal nutrition will take you months or even years to achieve. But the zest for living encouraged by a sustained blood-sugar level may be achieved immediately. Plan tomorrow to get from one-third to one-half of your daily protein at breakfast. A light lunch with its fair share of protein will help sustain you through the afternoon. A glass of milk and a cottage cheese and fruit salad is excellent.

"A habit cannot be tossed out the window," said Mark Twain. "It must be coaxed down the stairs—one step at a time." If it's your habit to slight breakfast, it may take a little while to develop good breakfast habits. For just one week try a high protein breakfast, a medium-sized lunch with adequate protein, and a light supper—and you may never again neglect breakfast. By avoiding the fuss of fixing a heavy evening meal, you and your family may have more time and energy for companionship and evening fun together.

Most books on nutrition emphasize that protein is expensive. This isn't necessarily so! Protein can be quite expensive if you insist on getting it from sirloin steak. A quart of milk made from nonfat skim milk powder gives you 49 per cent of your daily allowance for protein at a cost of only nine cents. You will find in Chapter 7 that skim milk may also be kinder to your arteries than the steak.

8. W. W. Tuttle, L. Daum, R. Larsen, J. Salzano, and L. Roloff, *Journal of the American Dietetic Association*, Vol. 30, p. 674, 1954.

Chapter 4

BODY-BUILDING PROTEIN

Now we're getting somewhere. We know that hour-to-hour get-up-and-go depends in part upon the energy-sustaining effect of protein on our blood sugar. We cannot talk about protein very long without getting into the subject of the chemical units from which protein is made. Just as bread is made from flour, water yeast, milk, and salt, the ingredients of protein are various amino acids. Twenty-two amino acids are known to be used by the body. Eight of these are essential and must be supplied by food. We're in trouble if they're not. If the other fourteen are not available in adequate amounts, our bodies can manufacture them from the eight essential amino acids.

You'll be running into their names occasionally so you'll want to be prepared to spot them as the essential amino acids that make up high quality protein: tryptophan, lysine, methionine, threonine, phenylalanine, leucine, isoleucine, and valine. There is evidence that two more amino acids, histidine and arginine, cannot be made by the body fast enough to meet the rapid growth needs of children. Here is a list of the other amino acids which, in case of shortage, you can produce in your

body from the eight essential amino acids: alanine, gly-
cine, glutamic acid, beta-hydroxyglutamic acid, aspartic
acid, cystine, cysteine, tyrosine, proline, hydroxyproline,
serine, and norleucine. Aren't we lucky that our bodies
know how to make these even though we can't pro-
nounce them!

Some pill purveyors try to take advantage of most
people's ignorance in nutritional matters by throwing
in a touch of protein powder and then adding a long
list of impressive-looking amino acids to the label. It
looks like you are getting a lot for your money unless
you know that they only supply about one two-hun-
dredths of your daily allowance of the various amino
acids. If a day's allowance of protein were put in a pill,
it would choke an elephant. Some stores offer protein
tablets or wafers, but they cannot compare in nutritional value with a glass of skim milk—and they are a
lot more expensive.

You'll recall that no body cells can be built without protein—but any old protein won't do. Just as a
chain is no stronger than its weakest link, a deficiency
of any of the eight essential amino acids will knock out
the body-building use of protein. Dr. Paul Cannon of
the University of Chicago fed rats four of the eight
essential amino acids at the beginning of the day and
the other four a few hours later. He found that the
amino acids don't lounge around waiting for the missing
ones to come along. For maintenance and growth, all
eight essential amino acids must be available at the same
time.

Protein foods (such as meat, fish, poultry, milk,
cheese, eggs, soybeans, and wheat germ) that contain
all of the eight essential amino acids in useful quantities
are called "complete." An incomplete protein such as
gelatin, which has almost no tryptophan (and is very
low in threonine, methionine, and isoleucine), cannot

by itself be used to build a body cell. However, when eaten with other complete proteins, it may be supplemented in a way that helps utilize it.

WHICH PROTEIN IS BEST?

The balance of the amino acids in a protein food determines its value for building new tissues and replacing old or damaged ones. Milk and eggs have the highest body-building values. This should be expected. These are the foods on which the young must survive during the first part of their life. Here is a list of protein-rich foods ranked according to their values for building new tissue: [1]

Food	Body-Building Value	Food	Body-Building Value
Milk, human	95	Whole wheat	67
Egg	94	Whole oats	66
Milk, cow	90	Barley	64
Corn germ, defatted	78	Dried brewer's yeast	63
Liver, animal	77	Cottonseed meal	62
Meat, beef	76	Corn, whole	60
Fish	76	Whole rye	58
Wheat germ	75	Peanuts	56
Soybeans	75	Dried peas and beans	40
Rice, whole	75		

You will note that peas and beans have a low body-building value. You must eat about twice as much of them to get the same benefit as with the more complete proteins such as eggs or milk. In other words, if you rely on proteins with a low body-building value, your protein total might have to be as high as 200 per cent

1. *Nutritional Data*, 4th ed., pp. 6-7. (Pittsburgh: H. J. Heinz Company, 1960.)

in order to get the same body-building effect that a total of 100 per cent would give you if you use the better balanced proteins of milk, eggs, meat, wheat germ or soybeans. By-products of milk such as cheese, nonfat skim milk, and yogurt have the same value as milk.

Other proteins with low body-building values are white flour, corn meal, corn grits and, in general, the proteins in fruits and vegetables. The sweet and white potato are exceptions—they do not contain much protein but what's there has a body-building value about equal to animal protein.

DOVETAILING YOUR PROTEINS

When you eat a varied diet, amino acids in various foods will often supplement each other. For example, if beans that are very low in methionine are eaten with bread that is very low in lysine, they will have a higher body-building value than when eaten separately. They will not, however, quite equal milk or meat. Milk and eggs, which have the highest values, are particularly valuable in supplementing the poorer proteins and raising their body-building values.

Fifteen college girls at the University of Nebraska volunteered for an experiment in which the supplementary value of milk protein was tested. For the first three weeks, their breakfasts had only proteins with low body-building value. This consisted of bread (made without milk), butter, jelly, fruit and coffee. For the noon and evening meal they had a good diet, which included one glass of milk at noon and two glasses of milk in the evening. In the second three weeks, the menu was the same except that one glass of milk was taken from the evening meal and added to the breakfast. You will note that the foods during both three-

week periods were exactly the same—the only difference was in the timing of the three daily glasses of milk.
Chemical studies showed that the girls built more girl
when milk was included at breakfast. This was due to
the generous supplies of the eight essential amino acids
in milk which supplemented the poor protein in the
white bread used at breakfast.[2]

Heat affects protein. The protein in beans is made
more digestible by cooking. Soybeans especially do not
achieve their high biological value until cooked. On the
other hand, the high heating of cereals (as in flaked or
puffed breakfast foods) and unusually high temperatures applied to meat or milk damage some of the amino
acids. Normal cooking does not materially affect meat
or milk.

2. Ruth M. Leverton, "Amino Acids," from *Food, The Yearbook
of Agriculture 1959*, p. 67. (Washington, D.C.: U.S. Government
Printing Office.)

Chapter 5

AN APPROACH TO OPTIMAL PROTEIN

The National Research Council was formed to make the combined talents of America's leading scientists available to the nation. They have formulated "Recommended Dietary Allowances" designed to keep the people of our nation in good health.[1] Their work has provided us with a scientific standard we can use in evaluating our food habits.

A unique feature of this book is a Food Table that shows the protein, vitamins, and minerals in various foods as a *percentage of the Council's recommended daily allowance* for a 25-year-old moderately active American man weighing 154 pounds. This percentage figure enables you to see at a glance the nutritional contribution that each food will make in your daily diet. The Food Table, which begins on page 217, is the very heart of this book. Without it you could not begin your journey toward optimal nutrition. Take a look at it right now and notice the type of information it gives you about each food. After you have looked at the Food Table, PLEASE TURN TO PAGE 189 AND NOTICE HOW YOU CAN USE THIS UNIQUE FOOD TABLE TO ADD UP THE TOTALS OF VARIOUS NUTRIENTS IN YOUR OWN DIET.

The National Research Council bases its protein

1. *Recommended Dietary Allowances, Revised 1958,* Publication 589. (Washington, D.C.: National Academy of Sciences—National Research Council, 1958.) This publication was revised in 1964.

allowance on your weight. When expressed in terms
of our Food Table, it recommends that both men
and women have a protein total of 6.5 per cent for
each ten pounds of weight. Here is a table that indicates
the daily protein total recommended for both men
and women:

Pounds	Recommended Protein Total	Pounds	Recommended Protein Total
90	59%	150	98%
100	65%	160	104%
110	72%	170	111%
120	78%	180	117%
130	85%	190	124%
140	91%	200	130%

Expectant mothers, nursing mothers, and growing children have greater protein needs for each pound
of body weight than the rest of us. To see the National
Research Council's recommendations for these people,
turn to the table on page 216. This table, entitled
"Recommended • Allowances for Various Groups,"
shows that during the second half of pregnancy the
protein total of a 128-pound woman should total 111
per cent. When a mother is nursing, her daily protein
total should be increased to 140 per cent. A seven- to
nine-year-old child needs more protein than the average
woman! Notice the heavy nutritional needs of teenagers. A boy of sixteen needs 143 per cent protein total,
a 175 per cent calcium total, and a 150 per cent iron
total. If Junior has been eating a lot lately, now you
know why.

ARE THESE ALLOWANCES OPTIMAL?

Dr. Robert Elman and Dr. Paul R. Cannon in analyzing these recommendations stated, "The difficulty with these allowances is, however, that they presumably apply to good protein, yet not all dietary protein is 'good' protein, particularly when a considerable proportion comes from overmilled or overprocessed foods, as, for example, white flour, corn grits, and toasted or puffed cereals." [2]

The allowances of the National Research Council are not necessarily optimal. Their allowances for our daily intake of protein, vitamins, and minerals have generally been arrived at by starting at the *minimum needed to avoid deficiency symptoms* and then adding a margin of safety above the minimum. The Council has clearly stated regarding their allowances, "Information available is not adequate to permit designation of these as optimal levels of intake." [3]

Dr. Sherman worked with the National Research Council, and some of their allowances are based on his work. "Nearly all current recommendations represent only a first step in the guidance of daily food habits by the newest knowledge of nutrition," according to Dr. Sherman. "For, nearly all current recommendations are still in some degree tradition-bound. Those who write them hesitate to advocate more than a slight adjustment of food habits in the direction indicated by our nutritional knowledge." [4]

At this point you may be wondering, "Well, why

2. Robert Elman and Paul R. Cannon, "Protein Malnutrition," from Norman Jolliffe, ed., *Clinical Nutrition*, p. 189. (New York: Hoeber Medical Division, Harper & Row, Publishers, Inc., 1950.)
3. *Recommended Dietary Allowances, Revised 1958, op. cit.,* p. 1.
4. Henry C. Sherman, *The Nutritional Improvement of Life,* p. 199. (New York: Columbia University Press, 1950.)

don't those fellows on the National Research Council come up with some optimal human recommendations?" I am sure the members of the board would like nothing better, for their silence on optimal human levels leaves a front yard in which unscientific food faddists can romp around. Here's why the Council can't do it.

THE DIFFICULTIES OF HUMAN RESEARCH

Through careful and inspired laboratory work, it is possible to experiment with various animals and gradually work toward a scientific knowledge of optimal nutrition for those animals. But, regretfully, such information will never be obtained for humans in our time. Experiments in optimal nutrition must cover the entire lifetime of many individuals and preferably it should extend to both previous and future generations. Is it possible to raise large numbers of humans under laboratory control for their entire lives? Year in and year out the only food they could have would be the experimental ration decreed by scientists. A single experiment would require an entire human lifetime, which could run between seventy and one hundred or more years, and hundreds of experiments would be necessary. Even if large numbers of cooperative humans could be found to submit to this sort of thing, the job of determining optimal human nutrition still couldn't be done in time to benefit you and me.

This is why the rat and other laboratory animals are relied upon so much in nutritional research. They are relatively inexpensive to maintain, and the normal lifetime of the rat is only one-thirtieth that of a human. One day in a rat's life thus equals one month of a human life for experimental purposes. Most experiments with humans run for two to twelve weeks. This is like testing a rat for one to three days. It's too short a time to draw final conclusions. Even if it were possible to use human beings for long-term optimal nutrition experiments, it would take many centuries to cover the laboratory work that has been done, for example, with rats on Sherman's Diets A and B.

Minimums are simpler. By eating a diet adequate except for a single nutrient, cooperative human volunteers may quickly show deficiency symptoms. Their blood may be low in this nutrient. Their reserve supply may be tapped. Their bodies may even start consuming themselves to meet this emergency. Thus scientists have found out a lot about human minimums—but we know precious little about human optimums.

AN APPROACH TO OPTIMAL NUTRITION

This puts us in a quandary. You and I need information on optimal nutrition right now—and we find that it may not be available for a thousand years, if then! We know more about nourishing mice, guinea pigs, and chickens than ourselves.

Some people have tried to solve this problem by using a heavy hand with all of the known nutrients on the theory that the body can get rid of any excess not needed. But Dr. Sherman cautions us, "It is easily conceivable that saturation . . . with some nutrients may be disadvantageous. Discrimination is extremely important. An undiscriminating openhandedness with all nutrients might be not only wasteful but also in some directions a handicap to the building of the highest health of which the individual is capable." [5]

The fallacy of an indiscriminate openhandedness becomes apparent when we realize that too much salt may bring on high blood pressure. Too much saturated fat in your diet may play a part in setting the stage

5. *Ibid.*, p. 157.

for a heart attack. Large excesses of vitamins A and D are highly toxic. A daily oversupply of calories (whether large or small) will cause you to gain weight and reduce your probable life span.

What can we do to work toward the optimal energy and health that Sherman has shown us is possible? As I see it, the intelligent course is to base our nutrition on the recommended allowances of the National Research Council. Then, using their recommendations as a starting point, we can tentatively vary the nutrients in our diet in the directions indicated by animal and human research. Such an approach yields no final answers, but it will launch us on a nutritional adventure that may pay off in many ways.

Optimal, you will recall, means avoiding too little or too much. The optimal level, then, *is the level at which you get the greatest benefits.*

The Food Table beginning on Page 217 gives you the protein contribution of foods that are frequently relied upon for their protein values:

Protein Food	Amount	% of Daily Protein Allowance
Almonds	14 almonds	4%
Beans, cooked kidney	½ cup	11%
Beans, cooked navy	½ cup	11%
Beef, dried chipped	2 ounces	27%
Bluefish, baked	3 ounces	31%
Bread, whole wheat	1 slice	3%
Cashew nuts, roasted	1 tablespoon	2%
Cheese, processed cheddar	1 ounce	10%
Cheese, creamed cottage	½ cup	21%
Chicken, fried leg	4.3 ounces	39%
Chile con carne with beans	1 cup	27%
Clams, raw without shell	3 ounces	16%
Codfish, cooked	3 ounces	25%
Crabmeat	3 ounces	20%
Hamburger, broiled lean	3 ounce patty	33%
Hotdog, including bun	1 hotdog	16%
Kidneys, cooked beef	3 ounces	35%
Lamb chop, broiled	1 chop	36%
Liver, fried beef	3 ounces	28%
Mackerel, broiled	3 ounces	27%

Protein Food	Amount	% of Daily Protein Allowance
Milk, buttermilk	1 cup	12%
Milk, chocolate	1 cup	11%
Milk, dry skim	1 tablespoon	3%
Milk, skim	1 cup	12%
Milk, skim	1 quart	49%
Milk, whole	1 cup	12%
Oatmeal	½ cup	4%
Oysters, raw	8 medium	14%
Peanuts	1 ounce	11%
Pecans	1 tablespoon	1%
Perch, ocean fried breaded	3 ounces	23%
Sausage, Vienna canned	3 ounces	19%
Soup, cream of mushroom	1 cup	10%
Soybean curd (tofu)	4.2 ounces	12%
Soybeans, dried cooked	½ cup	16%
Soybean flour	1 cup	53%
Soybeans, cooked green	½ cup	11%
Soybean milk	1 cup	11%
Soybean sprouts	½ cup	5%
Steak, sirloin	3 ounces	29%
Tuna, canned	3 ounces	36%
Turkey, cooked	3 ounces	29%
Wheat germ	½ cup	12%
Yeast, torula	1 tablespoon	6%
Yogurt, commercial	½ cup	6%

Chapter 6

THE FAT OF THE LAND

Since 1900 the life expectancy of Americans has increased. But don't be too smug about it because an increase in overall life expectancy may not apply to you—yet. Most of the increase has come from the lowering of the death rate of children under five years and through the control of infectious diseases. The older folks aren't getting their fair share of added life, and the food they eat may be largely responsible.[1]

As our standard of living has increased over the years, we have chosen diets that in some ways produce greater amounts of disease. The U.S. Department of Agriculture has recently pointed out that "As early as 1904, an increase of 40 per cent was observed in diseases of the circulatory apparatus and kidneys and a 15 per cent increase in cancer in one generation. In the 1930's during the depression, autopsies of poorly nourished bodies revealed little fatty clogging of the arteries." The war, which imposed food restrictions on peoples throughout the world, "slackened the mortality rates from diabetes and other metabolic disorders as well as

1. *Food, The Yearbook of Agriculture 1959*, Department of Agriculture, p. 5. (Washington, D.C.: U.S. Government Printing Office.)

from cardiovascular diseases. The trends reversed after the war to accelerated rates . . . cardiovascular diseases rose rapidly to top place as the reported cause of deaths in the United States." [2]

Compelling evidence now shows that our bodies are ill equipped to handle the heavy loads of fat that are being swallowed today. Before 1900 most folks got about 31 per cent of their calories from fat. In the middle 1930's this had risen to about 37 per cent, and by the middle 1950's this jumped to about 43 per cent! Unfortunately, this increase in the use of fats has been paralleled by an increase in the rate of coronary heart attacks.

Your body is extremely limited in its ability to store protein and carbohydrate, but it is almost unlimited (alas!) in its ability to store fat. Each pound of fatty tissue that you store constitutes an energy reserve of about 3,500 calories.[3] Regardless of whether you overeat in protein, carbohydrate, or fat, *everything above your needs is stored as fat*—usually where you want it least.

USES OF FAT

In the past, fats have been associated with luxury; they were a symbol of prosperity and hospitality, as when the fatted calf was prepared for merrymaking. Fat adds a flavoring and consistency to food that is deeply satisfying. It is also a concentrated source of energy. An ounce of pure carbohydrate, such as sugar, contains about 110 calories; an ounce of pure protein contains about the same number of calories; but an

2. *Ibid.*, p. 81.
3. Michael G. Wohl, "Obesity," from Michael G. Wohl and Robert S. Goodhart, eas., *Modern Nutrition in Health and Disease*, p. 865. (Philadelphia: Lea & Febiger, 1960.)

ounce of fat contains more than twice as many calories! This makes it most useful in case you plan to explore the North Pole. Until then, however, your road to optimal nutrition should take the short cut through fatland.

Even so, fats have an important part to play in your body. One nice thing we can say about fat is that its characteristic distribution enables the profiles of men and women to develop such charming differences. About half of your fat is deposited under your skin where it acts as an insulator to protect your body from extremes in temperature. Cushions of fat stored around your vital internal organs help to protect them from bumps and knocks. If you reduce weight too rapidly, they may come in contact with each other and be critically injured.

Small amounts of fat have many jobs to do in your body. Fat plays an important part in the production of sex hormones. In addition to making you masculine or feminine, these hormones help to regulate your body. Fat also is needed for the production of bile. When this vital digestive enzyme is deficient, you'll have trouble digesting foods containing fat. Fats are needed to carry vitamins A, D, E, and K into your blood. Certain minerals such as calcium may be poorly absorbed if not accompanied by a small amount of fat. A tiny speck of fat is bound into the structure of each cell when it is formed from protein. This fat is locked in and cannot be withdrawn to meet the body's energy needs in case of starvation.

Dr. George O. Burr of the University of Minnesota has warned us that when fats get rancid they destroy the fat-soluble vitamins.[4] Vitamin E is espe-

4. George O. Burr, "The Role of Fat in the Diet," from Michael G. Wohl, ed., *Dietotherapy, Clinical Application of Modern Nutrition,* p. 79. (Philadelphia: W. B. Saunders Company, 1945.)

cially sensitive and may be completely wiped out by rancid fat. If mayonnaise, butter, ham, or salad oil smell even faintly rancid, *throw them out*. Be on the lookout for rancid nuts displayed in heated cases and rancid popcorn that has not been freshly popped. A food like wheat germ that contains a natural oil should be refrigerated. Keeping a can of bacon drippings near the stove may be doubly unwise—they get rancid easily and they will add to your intake of undesirable saturated fat.

SATURATED *VS.* UNSATURATED FATS

Recent research has shown that solid *saturated* fats (as in meat or butter) and liquid *unsaturated* fats (as in corn oil or cottonseed oil) may behave differently in your body. Unfortunately, the solid saturated fats may play a large part in our heavy death rate in coronary heart disease. Unsaturated liquid fats may counteract some of the undesirable effects of solid fats. It is, then, important that we get on a first-name basis with these two types of fat so that we can spot them easily.

Saturated fats, in general, come from animals. Coconut oil is one of the few exceptions. They are called "saturated" because they are saturated with all the hydrogen atoms they can hold and there is no room for more hangers-on. Liquid oils or unsaturated fats, on the other hand, have room for additional hydrogen atoms to be attached. In the process called "hydrogenation," extra hydrogen atoms are attached to unsaturated vegetable oils. This changes these oils into a solid shortening or margarine that is more saturated.

Here is where to look for these two types of fat:

Food with Large Amounts of Saturated Fats	Food with Large Amounts of Unsaturated Fats
Whole milk	Corn oil such as Mazola
Cream	Cottonseed oil such as Wesson oil
Butter	Olives and olive oil
Ice cream	Safflower oil
Cheese (except cottage cheese)	Sunflower oil
Beef	Soybean oil
Pork	Peanut oil
Bacon	Other vegetable oils
Lamb	Nuts
Poultry	Peanuts
Sausage	Peanut butter when not hydrogenated
Coconut oil	Soybeans
Margarine	Avocados
Lard	Fish oils
Hydrogenated vegetable shortenings	Fatty fish (such as tuna or mackerel)
Peanut butter when hydrogenated	Salad dressings such as mayonnaise, French dressing, etc.
Chocolate	
Eggs	
Liverwurst and other luncheon meats	
Hot dogs	

You will note in our Food Table that there are three columns dealing with calories. The first one gives the calories of saturated fat in each food. The middle column shows the total fat calories supplied by *both saturated and unsaturated fats*. The third column shows the *total calories* from protein, carbohydrates, and fats. You will notice that chicken has less saturated fat than beef. Trimming the outside fat from steak and roasts will reduce your intake of saturated fat. Selecting leaner cuts such as round steak also helps. When cottage cheese is made, almost all of the saturated butterfat is removed. Since it is almost fat-free, it is an extremely useful food for one interested in optimal nutrition. A small amount of fat is added when cottage cheese is creamed. Recently, margarine makers have developed ways to minimize the effects of hydrogenation. Some margarines, such as Emdee, Mazola, and Fleischmann's, now contain more unsaturated fats than butter or the usual margarine.

You will find that milk is a great help in achieving optimal levels of protein, B₂, and calcium. In whole milk, half of the calories are in the form of butterfat—which unfortunately is largely saturated. Skim milk or buttermilk, on the other hand, contain almost no fat. So don't let your concern over fat lead you to cut out milk or you're taking one step backward to offset an important forward step. Switch to buttermilk or skim milk fortified with vitamin D. In some foods the saturated fat is visible and you can avoid it to some extent. But like a snake in the grass, it may be hidden. Only about one-third to one-half of the fat in foods can be seen. You'll have to rely on the Food Table to warn you about the invisible fat. Any foods with a greasy or oily texture are guaranteed to be teeming with it.

LINOLEIC ACID

The nutritional spotlight has now been turned on linoleic acid, the most important of the unsaturated fats. Don't think of this as an acid like vinegar—it occurs in foods as a bland fat that is practically tasteless. Linoleic acid means a great deal to you in your quest for optimal nutrition. Scientists have been prying into its private affairs and have found that it may play an important part in preventing coronary attacks. Dr. Ancel Keys has found that a little over two parts of linoleic acid may offset the possible artery-clogging effect of one part of saturated fat.

This nutrient is essential for the development of a beautiful skin for babies. Human milk contains two to four times more linoleic acid than cow's milk. About five per cent of the calories in human milk come from linoleic acid. Babies who are not adequately supplied with linoleic acid develop scaly, itchy skin that can break out into sores when scratched.

A man who works for me once told me that he was unable to sleep because the four young children next door were broken out literally from head to toe with painful sores that kept them crying during the night. When I talked with their desperate father, I found that he had taken them to two clinics and that both shots and ointments had brought no relief. Knowing that harassed and overloaded doctors sometimes overlook nutritional factors, I inquired into the children's diet and found that ignorance of nutrition had permitted the children to select for themselves a diet made up largely of candy, soft drinks, crackers, and desserts. I told the father to discontinue medications and give each child two tablespoons of corn oil each day. I also suggested that each child drink a quart of powdered skim milk to provide an economical source of protein for rapid healing. This therapy cost approximately ten cents per child per day.

When I went to see these children ten days later, it almost seemed as if a miracle had taken place. They were smiling and happy, and not one child could find even one sore to show me. The healing had been so complete that it took quite a bit of searching for the children to find scars where the sores had been. Three years later there had been no recurrence.

Research has shown that an infant may get too fat if he does not get enough fat in the form of linoleic acid. Doctors fed infants on diets with various amounts of linoleic acid.[5] In some diets this essential fat was almost absent; in others, it furnished up to eight per cent of the total calories. They found that when linoleic acid was adequately supplied, the infants usually decreased their caloric intake. When linoleic acid was withdrawn and replaced with another fat, they ate significantly more. Flabby fat in infants is as undesirable as in adults, even though it looks cuter on a smiling baby. This research indicated that overeating may in part be associated with failure to provide a growing child with nutrients it requires.

Many women who want lovely skin and hair try to achieve them by applying expensive creams and lotions. The loveliest skin and hair are inside jobs. They come naturally when the blood supplying your skin is richly supplied with the nutrients required by your body. Linoleic acid is particularly needed for that attractive glow of health. Outside applications of expensive creams are not even a poor substitute for this important nutrient.

Often skin troubles that resist medical treatment are cured when nutrition is improved. Frank S. developed sores in his scalp that for over a year defied various doctors. His inflamed scalp itched terribly night and day, and the entire back of his head had a skullcap of scabs. For months I pleaded with him to improve his nutrition, but this approach was not for him. Hope rose anew with each new doctor he saw. The idea that his trouble was associated with nutrition seemed ridiculous both to him and his doctors. One year, four doctors (including a dermatologist), much pain, and many

5. D. J. D. Adam, A. E. Hansen, and Hilda F. Wiese, *Journal of Nutrition,* Vol. 66, p. 555, 1958.

dollars later, he finally agreed to use daily two table-spoons of corn oil plus two heaping tablespoons of yeast (a concentrated source of B vitamins), along with his medication. Within thirty days, his scalp was well on its way toward healing. In forty-five days—no sores at all! I wish more doctors realized that their therapy works best when accompanied by excellent nutrition!

Your dog or cat can also benefit from your interest in nutrition. An adequate supply of unsaturated vege-table oil in his diet will help him develop a beautiful sleek coat. Sometimes eczema in animals will respond rapidly to a diet adequate in linoleic fat. One house-wife whose dog had been annoyed with eczema for a long time told me that it cleared up in about a week. "A tablespoon of oil a day is a lot cheaper than a visit to the vet," she added.

The best sources of linoleic acid are oils pressed from seeds, grains, and nuts. Safflower oil is tops with a total of 72 per cent linoleic acid. The remaining 28 per cent consists of oleic acid (another unsaturated fat) and small amounts of saturated fatty acids. Here is the linoleic acid content of other oils: sunflower oil 70 per cent, corn oil 57 per cent, soybean oil 55 per cent, wheat germ oil 50 per cent, cottonseed oil 47 per cent, peanut oil 29 per cent, pecan oil 20 per cent. I was sorry to find that perhaps the most delicious of the oils—olive oil—has only 10 per cent linoleic acid. Although poultry has a predominantly saturated fat, it contains 23 per cent linoleic acid. The fats in pork, lard, shortening, regular margarine, lamb, butter, and the fat of beef all contain less than 10 per cent. Mazola-type margarines contain 22 per cent linoleic acid and should therefore be preferred to the regular margarines.

One or two tablespoons of vegetable oil each day will provide your body with a generous supply of linoleic acid. This may be added to meat loaves, stews, breads, or other dishes or taken in the form of salad dressings such as mayonnaise or French dressing.

Mineral oil is sometimes used for frying, salad dressings, or as a laxative. It absorbs fat-soluble vitamins and thus may deprive you of your full quota of these essential nutrients. Medical journals have repeatedly warned against its use.

Most books on nutrition speak of three essential fatty acids: linoleic acid, linolenic acid, and arachidonic acid. Our search for optimal nutrition need not be complicated by the last two. Research indicates that linolenic acid is not essential and you can make your own arachidonic acid in your body if you are well supplied with linoleic acid.

In the next chapter we will discuss how your arteries may be corroded by the high-fat American diet. Since coronary heart attacks are a leading cause of death among Americans today, it is urgent that we work toward optimal levels of fat in our diet.

Chapter 7

FATS CAN BE DANGEROUS

Research of the last decade has shown that, for optimal nutrition, we must not only get enough fat in our diet but we must also be careful not to get too much. Oversupply seems to be far more dangerous than undersupply. In 1955 in the United States, slightly over one-fourth of all deaths were caused by blockage of the coronary arteries upon which the heart is solely dependent for its blood supply. This is nearly twice the toll of all cancers, which is the second leading cause of death. It is almost nine times the deaths caused by auto accidents. In many other countries, coronary heart disease is a minor problem. In some "primitive" areas this disease is almost unknown! It tends to be associated with prosperity. And you're prosperous enough to run the risk of getting it.

Let's see how the fats in your diet may lead to the development of a blod clot or a blockage that can shut off the blood supply to your heart. After you eat a meal with a lot of fat, little droplets of fat are absorbed into your blood and give it a milky appearance. Your liver gradually gathers these droplets from the blood and stores them temporarily until they are taken to the cells that burn them for energy or to your fat bulges that store them. Cholesterol is one of the porters used in moving fat from the liver. When you eat large amounts of fat, your body needs more cholesterol to move it around.

When cholesterol picks up a bit of fat in your liver and carries it, let's say, to the cells of your big toe, it then heads back to the liver. The arterial and venous network of your blood vessels is so complicated that it may wander around for hours before it gets back there. Thus, when you eat a high-fat diet, you may have a great deal of circulating cholesterol. Unfortunately, over a period of many years, some of this may get stuck in the lining of your arteries and gradually narrow the opening—somewhat as pipes are gradually clogged up by mineral deposits.

SCARRED ARTERIES

Cholesterol deposited in your coronary arteries not only tends to diminish their blood-carrying capacity, but it also has an important effect on the health of the artery itself. When cholesterol sticks to your arteries, the cells in the artery walls become crowded and poorly nourished. Connective tissue will tend to grow around these cholesterol patches to seal them off. Sooner or later some of the cells in the artery actually die and make tiny areas of ulceration on the inside. Your body will heal this, but unfortunately more scar tissue is formed that still further chokes off the blood supply to the cells in the walls of your coronary arteries. All of this roughens up the inside of your arteries and seriously constricts the flow of blood. After years of gradual deterioration, your vital coronary arteries may be so scarred up that the blood flow is cut way down. But the blood still oozes through. Then the axe falls.

"After a fatty meal the red cells in the blood may tend to stick together," say Dr. Ancel Keys, "and some tests show that the blood clots more readily than before." [1] When a blood clot forms and gets stuck in your coronary arteries, you're in trouble.

Usually when a heart attack comes, it does not block off the blood to all of the muscles of the heart. If it only affects a minor portion, your body can repair the damage in a few weeks of bed rest. If it is more serious, it can permanently impair your activity. If it is more serious yet, you will not survive the heart attack.

A few years ago, doctors noted that men with coronary attacks usually had high cholesterol levels. It seemed, at the time, reasonable to infer that cholesterol by itself was the culprit. Low-cholesterol diets were advised for many folks whose blood analysis showed high levels of cholesterol. However, your body makes four to six times more cholesterol than you probably get in your diet. In the words of detective fiction, cholesterol was implicated because it was found at the scene of the crime. Further evidence, however, indicated that it had partners in crime. It became apparent that since cholesterol is made by the body to do the job of transporting fat from the liver, it was only an accomplice. Other guilty parties are too much saturated fat and too much total fat.

Doctors during the Korean War noticed that the arteries of young American soldiers frequently contained large deposits of cholesterol—they call it atherosclerosis. Young Chinese and Korean soldiers, when autopsied, had little or no atherosclerosis. Since that time, scientists have compared the arteries of many

1. Ancel and Margaret Keys, *Eat Well and Stay Well*. Copyright © 1959, 1963 by Ancel and Margaret Keys. Reprinted by permission of Doubleday & Company, Inc.

people throughout the world. They have found, for
example, that the Japanese in Japan have very little
atherosclerosis because they have very little fat in their
diet. The Japanese in Hawaii have more dietary fat
and more atherosclerosis. The Japanese living in California who eat large amounts of saturated fat have done
just as good a job of corroding their arteries as other
Americans.

LOWERING YOUR CHOLESTEROL

The *unsaturated* fats listed on page 45 do not tend
to raise the cholesterol level in the blood and may even
lower it. Dr. Ancel Keys has found that a little over
two parts of linoleic acid may offset the cholesterol-
raising effect of one part of saturated fat.[2] This was
good news to the corn oil boys.

Hard regular physical exercise may help hold down
your cholesterol level. But a few pushups in the morning
won't knock out much cholesterol for you. Dr. Keys
says, "Physiologically, there does not seem to be much
prospect of achieving anything significant unless the
exercise is hard enough or long enough, or both, to
give the heart and circulation some real work to do
and to add up to an appreciable number of calories
burned, say at least 2,000 *extra* calories a week." [3] All
you have to do to use up 2,000 extra calories is to walk
for fourteen hours, or waltz for about ten hours, or
play the cello for twenty-two hours!

This problem of saturated *versus* unsaturated fat,
how the blood clots in damaged arteries, and the inter-
play of various factors in the formation of death-dealing
or crippling coronary blockages is being given top

2. A. Keys, J. T. Anderson, and F. Grande, "Serum Cholesterol
in Man: Diet Fat and Intrinsic Responsiveness," *Circulation*, Vol. 19,
p. 201, 1959.
3. Ancel and Margaret Keys, *op. cit.*, p. 38.

priority in many research laboratories today. Dietary cholesterol, tension, lack of exercise, and other factors may play a direct or indirect part. But enough of the jigsaw has been put together to indicate practical things that we can do now to greatly lessen our chances of a coronary attack. The amount and kind of fat in our diet is not the only factor in avoiding a coronary. It is, however, a prime factor and it is one that we can most easily control.

THE ANTI-CORONARY CLUB

In the spring of 1957, the late Dr. Norman Jolliffe, Director of the Board of Nutrition of the Department of Health, City of New York, formed the Anti-Coronary Club to determine the effects of a prudent diet on the cholesterol levels of middle-aged men. He called for volunteers who would be willing to follow the recommended diet until they reached the age of sixty-five. He had no difficulty getting them. Before they made any dietary changes, several cholesterol tests were taken over a period of one to three months to accurately determine the original cholesterol level of these men.

Each was given the following instructions designed to lower the total fat intake and to insure adequate amounts of linoleic acid:

1. Consume adequate amounts of high-grade protein at each meal. The sources for these include: cottage-type cheese, fat-free milk, chicken, turkey, veal, leaner cuts of beef, mutton, lamb, and pork (with the visible fat removed), fish, seafood, and egg whites.
Remember there are 21 meals each week. Therefore, from this list, include fresh or canned fish or seafood at least five times each week. Do

not be limited to the leaner fish but include fat fish as well, as they are good sources of polyunsaturated fatty acids. Bake, roast, broil, or boil meats and poultry. Fish may be fried as instructed. Serve beef, lamb, mutton, and veal medium to well done: when rare, less fat drains off. When fat is required in food preparation, use a high linoleic acid oil or an 80 per cent unaltered high linoleic acid margarine or cooking fat. Use veal or fowl four meals each week or oftener. Use beef, lamb, mutton, or pork not oftener than four times each week. For the other eight meals each week use cottage-type cheese or egg whites. Unless instructed otherwise, you may include four egg yolks each week. You may also use whole milk for coffee but otherwise restrict the use of milk to nonfat varieties such as fresh or reconstituted skim milk, fat-free buttermilk, or evaporated skim milk. When instructed, you may add an emulsion of corn oil to your skim milk.

2. Consume a minimum of 1 ounce of corn oil, or its equivalent, at the table each day exclusive of that used in food preparation. This may be added to milk, cereals, or desserts, or an 80 per cent unaltered corn oil margarine used as a table spread. When fats are desired in cooking or baking, use corn oil or a specially prepared equivalent.

3. Do not eat the following except under unusual circumstances: butter, ordinary (partially hydrogenated) margarine and shortenings, lard, or cream or foods containing them in large amounts such as most cakes and pastries. In place of butter and margarine, use an 80 per cent unaltered corn oil margarine; in place of shortening use either corn oil or a specially prepared 80 per cent unaltered corn oil margarine; in place of cream use an emulsion of corn oil.

4. Balance your diet by consuming adequate

amounts of bread, cereals, nuts, vegetables, and fruits.[4]

Overweight men were instructed to use this same food pattern but no fat of any kind was to be added in cooking or used at the table. This reducing diet provides about 1,600 calories.

The prudent diet recommended by Dr. Jolliffe for the members of the Anti-Coronary Club has a protein total of 186 per cent to 214 per cent. The total fat calories amounted to 17 per cent to 20 per cent of the total calories. Saturated fat ran 7 per cent to 8 per cent of the total calories. These diets contain 2,000 to 2,700 calories depending upon the size and activity of the men.

The cholesterol tests made before the men adopted the prudent diet were found to average 250 milligrams per 100 cubic centimeters of blood in the 50- to 59-year-old group. After six months on this diet, the average cholesterol of the group had fallen from 250 to 222 milligrams per 100 cc. Dr. Jolliffe did not regard this diet as optimal. He has, however, demonstrated that a prudent change in your diet can begin to lower your cholesterol level.

YOUR CHOLESTEROL LEVEL

No known diet will remove cholesterol deposits you now have. But by achieving a diet that has optimal fat levels, you should be able to keep these deposits from growing to the point where they cut off the blood supply to your heart.

Most Americans 40 years old living on an ordinary

4. Norman Jolliffe, Seymour H. Rinzler, and Morton Archer, "The Anti-Coronary Club; Including a Discussion of the Effects of a Prudent Diet on the Serum Cholesterol Level of Middle-Aged Men," *American Journal of Clinical Nutrition*, Vol. 7, p. 454, 1959.

diet will have between 220 and 270 milligrams of cholesterol in 100 cc. of blood serum. Some will go over
300 milligrams—I wouldn't want to write their insurance. There are a fortunate few with a value of less
than 200. Most physicians today feel that 225 milligrams
of cholesterol per 100 cc. should be considered as a
warning, and above 250 is definitely undesirable. If you
are under thirty years old, these limits should be set
25 to 30 points lower. In other countries that have
very little heart disease, most cholesterol values are not
over 200 *even in middle-aged men.* Your interest in
optimal nutrition may lead you to choose a goal of
under 200 milligrams of cholesterol per 100 cc. of
blood. Your doctor can assist you in getting a cholesterol test.

Dr. Clarence Cohn has found that our habit of
eating three square meals a day may tend to increase
our blood cholesterol. His research indicates we may
have lower cholesterol levels in addition to other health
benefits if we divide our daily food intake into about
eight small snacks. These snacks should be as nutritious
as the meals they are replacing, and must not run us
over our daily calorie budget.[5] I realize that this may
be difficult. The lion-size breakfast, squirrel-size lunch,
and bird-like supper may better fit most people's pattern
of living. I have tried this snacking technique for over
a year and I am convinced that, for me, it is a part of
optimal nutrition. As mentioned in Chapter 2, snacking
in place of meal-eating may help you control your
weight.

According to Dr. Keys, "Most populations that
seem to have relatively little coronary disease live on
diets that are rather high in leafy vegetables and fruits

5. Clarence Cohn, "Meal-Eating, Nibbling, and Body Metabolism," *Journal of the American Dietetic Association,* Vol. 38, pp
433-436, 1961.

as well as being low in sugar and in meat and dairy fats. Experiments with diets of this kind indicate that some part of their cholesterol-lowering action cannot be explained solely by the amounts of fat in the diet." [6] Recent research suggests that some of this effect may be due to the pectin (the substance that makes jellies jell) that is present in most fruits and berries. Pectin is especially concentrated in apples, citrus fruits, and fruits and berries that are noted for their value in making jellies. In citrus fruits most of the pectin is in the white inner rind and the pulp. It is lost when these fruits are juiced. To get the maximum food value from citrus fruits, you should eat the entire fruit except for the hull and seeds.[7]

AN APPROACH TO OPTIMAL FAT

The National Research Council offers no recommended allowances for fat. Dr. Ancel Keys, based on his extensive world-wide research, recommends that you get around 25 per cent of your calories from fat. He further suggests that the saturated fat calories be held to about 6 per cent of your total calories.[8]

"Some people are terrible at counting calories—and have the figures to prove it," said a wit. However, if you wish to follow Dr. Keys' recommendation, you can use the calorie values shown in the Food Table to work toward this balance in your diet. The Nutrition Analysis Form explained in Chapter 19 will make it easier to do.

6. Ancel and Margaret Keys, *op. cit.*, pp. 24–25.
7. Ancel Keys, Francisco Grande, and Joseph T. Anderson, "Fiber and Pectin in the Diet and Serum Cholesterol Concentration in Man," *Proceedings of the Society for Experimental Biology and Medicine*, Vol. 106, pp. 555-558, 1961.
8. Ancel and Margaret Keys, *op. cit.*, p. 46.

LIVING THE LOW-FAT LIFE

You can achieve the low-fat life if you are willing to apply your intelligence and ingenuity to the problem. Check the Food Table to see which foods run up your proportion of saturated fat and gradually cut down on these foods. You can give your butcher fair warning that you won't be needing many sirloin steaks, but be sure to tell him to have lots of fish and poultry in stock. Remember that if at first you don't succeed— you're running about average. If you keep trying to develop new food patterns, you may find that you will enjoy your food just as much as ever—possibly more so, because you'll have the added satisfaction of knowing that it may add more years to your life and more life to your years.

The more determined you are to work toward an optimal fat intake, the easier you will find it gradually becomes. (Remember that "optimal" doesn't necessarily mean an increased amount—it means the best level for your health.) There is a low-calorie French dressing that contains only 3 per cent of the calories that French dressing usually provides. Livestock is usually raised in a way that gives a very high fat content. For steak to be graded as prime, it must be heavily marbled with fat. As a nutrition-wise consumer, you may wish to demand leaner steaks from your butcher. They can grow them that way if consumers insist. You can learn many delicious ways to fix cottage cheese, and there are a number of excellent low-fat, low-calorie cookbooks to help you.* When you begin thinking of foods in terms of the amount of saturated fat they offer, you will discover many surprising things. Did you know that 62 per cent of the calories in ham-

* See pages 208-210.

burger consist of fat? It will help if you have your hamburger ground from lean meat from which all visible fat has been trimmed off first.

WHAT ABOUT OTHERS?

I suggest that you avoid forcing your program of optimal nutrition on others, no matter how much you love them. No one likes to be pushed around and most folks resent having their childhood food patterns altered. A "dietribe" at each meal will not have the effect you desire. When other people see the many benefits you are getting from your interest in optimal nutrition, they will begin to ask you what you are doing. They may envy your extra energy, finer appearance, and— what's even better—your improved disposition. And they probably won't let you get too far ahead of them. The new you will speak for itself.

Chapter 8

TOWARD OPTIMAL CARBOHYDRATES

Dr. Weston A. Price, a member of the Research Commission of the American Dental Association, spent his vacations for many years traveling throughout the world comparing the teeth of folks on primitive diets with those who relied on the civilized man's food. Dr. Ernest Hooten of Harvard said of his research, "Since we have known for a long time that savages have excellent teeth and that civilized men have terrible teeth, it seems to me that we have been extraordinarily stupid in concentrating all of our attention upon the task of finding out why our teeth are so poor, without ever bothering to learn why savage teeth are good. Dr. Weston Price seems to be the only person who possesses the scientific horse sense to supplement his knowledge of the probable causes of dental disease with a study of the dietary regimens which are associated with dental health." [1]

Dr. and Mrs. Price traveled to isolated villages in the Swiss Alps and compared the teeth of people there with relatives who lived in the cities of Switzerland.

1. Weston A. Price, *Nutrition and Physical Degeneration*, p. xvii. (Los Angeles: The American Academy of Applied Nutrition, 1948.)

They studied Eskimos in Alaska, many Indian groups throughout North and South America, Polynesians in the South Pacific, and tribes in Africa. Wherever they went throughout the globe, they found the same story. When these remote groups ate natural fruits, vegetables, and meats they had raised themselves, their teeth were almost free of decay—even though they used no toothbrushes and had particles of food stuck between their teeth a great deal of the time. When examining the teeth of people in many remote villages, Dr. Price noticed that some had cavities that had started but did not progress. It invariably turned out that they had gone to work somewhere else and for a time had eaten refined carbohydrates such as white flour, white polished rice, candy, cookies, cakes, soda pop, etc.

When studying several hundred skulls taken from burial mounds of Seminole Indians in Southern Florida, Dr. Price found ". . . the incidence of tooth decay was so low as to constitute an immunity of apparently 100 per cent, since in several hundred skulls not a single tooth was found to have been attacked by tooth decay." [2] He also examined the teeth of modern Seminoles who were living in the Florida swamps out of contact with modern civilization. "While their hunting territory had been grossly encroached upon by the white hunters," said Dr. Price, "they were still able to maintain a very high degree of physical excellence and high immunity to dental caries. Only four teeth in each hundred examined were found to have been attacked by tooth decay." He then examined Indians who lived in tourist attractions in nearby Miami who had adopted the diet of the white man. "Forty out of every hundred teeth examined," reported Dr. Price, "were found to have been attacked by tooth decay. . . ." Apparently the high intake of refined carbohydrates was responsible

2. *Ibid.*, p. 93.

for the *ten-times increase in tooth decay* among these Seminole Indians.

IT MAY TASTE GOOD, BUT—

Dr. Price's research indicates that our teeth will stay in good condition if we eat fresh natural foods. Unfortunately, when many foods are refined or processed, their carbohydrate content jumps to a point that defeats our natural defenses against decay. The term "carbohydrate" includes both sugars and starches. Fresh fruits such as bananas, figs, sweet cherries, and grapes are only 15 per cent carbohydrate. White potatoes are 19 per cent carbohydrate and even sweet potatoes only run 28 per cent. Other starchy vegetables such as fresh peas, beans, and sweet corn are only 16 per cent to 20 per cent carbohydrate. And vegetables such as carrots, onions, and turnips are only 10 per cent.

But look what happens when we refine some foods. Syrups run 60 to 74 per cent carbohydrate; jams, jellies and preserves are 65 to 71 per cent; and candies are 60 to 95 per cent. Bread is 46 to 60 per cent, and cakes and cookies go as high as 75 per cent. White sugar is almost 100 per cent carbohydrate!

Tooth decay is caused by lactic acid and other acids made by bacteria in your mouth. If this acid is strong enough, it attacks and dissolves the calcium in the enamel of your teeth. The Caries Control Laboratory at Ohio State University found that caries do not form in men or animals unless starch or sugar residues remain on the teeth long enough to stimulate the acid-forming bacteria. These acid-forming bacteria increase by the millions when carbohydrates stick in the crevices of your teeth. Your teeth just are not designed to survive the acid jackhammers of the teeming bacteria that suddenly multiply when you eat refined carbohydrates.

HOW MUCH SUGAR DO YOU USE?

During digestion all carbohydrates must be broken down into a simple sugar that can go directly into your blood. You may feel that you don't use much sugar— just a little in your coffee and on your cereal. But like an iceberg, the greater part is beneath the surface. One or more tablespoons are usually hiding in canned fruits, soft drinks, some fruit juices, bread, ice cream, Manhattans, and many highballs. A single large cookie or small candy bar can supply a half-ounce sugar. Jam, jelly, cakes, pies, puddings, custards, and gelatin desserts are loaded with it. You may be eating one or more cups of granulated white sugar each day without realizing it. Alcohol also contains empty carbohydrate calories.

Dr. Henry Sherman has warned us against this trend toward "empty calories." "The per capita consumption of sugar per year in the United States," said Dr. Sherman, "increased from about ten pounds in the 1820's to about one hundred pounds in the 1920's and most of the time since. The *difference* between the level of sugar consumption of our generation and that of four generations ago probably covers at least one-tenth of our total food calorie intake, and correspondingly displaces the equivalent of one tenth of all nutrients other than carbohydrate. . . ." [3]

THE SWEET TOOTH

The problem of the "sweet tooth" has led Dr. Hazel N. Hauck of the New York State College of Home

3. Reprinted with permission of The Macmillan Company from *Chemistry of Food and Nutrition* by Henry C. Sherman. Eighth edition Copyright 1952 by The Macmillan Company.

Economics to advise that we "choose our calories by the nutritional company they keep." The Vitamin-Mineral Index in our Food Table may offer a clue as to whether you're eating a food with somewhat empty calories or one that will do its fair share in helping you build the highest possible level of health. If a food has a Vitamin-Mineral Index of 0 or 1, you will note that, in most cases, the hand of man has increased the carbohydrate content and eliminated some of its natural health-building values.

Unfortunately, many mothers unwittingly develop a sweet tooth in their children from the cradle onward by putting sugar into the baby's formula. This can produce flabby butterballs that have the appearance of health, but doctors will tell you that overweight children are not so healthy as their leaner companions. Many foods are sweetened by their own sugars. For example, young peas and corn are sweeter than mature peas and corn. On the other hand, an immature banana is largely starchy but becomes sweeter as it ripens. Dr. A. E. Harper of the University of Wisconsin suggests that we use the natural sweetening available in fruits and vegetables to satisfy the "sweet tooth." Instead of cookies, keep fruit handy. Instead of soda pop, use orange or grape juice.

FOR EFFICIENT DIGESTION

The digestion of carbohydrates begins in the mouth. When food is thoroughly chewed, saliva (which contains a digestive enzyme) can begin the job of breaking it down into simple sugars which the body can use. Sometimes flatulence (intestinal gas) or colic can result when food is not properly chewed. When undigested food goes into the large bowel, it may contain some unabsorbed sugars which are fermented by bacteria that are lurking there. This fermentation can produce carbon dioxide, methane, and other gases in quantities that can be unpleasant.[4]

When most of your carbohydrate foods are selected from fresh fruits, vegetables, and whole-grain cereals, you will be getting desirable bulk in addition to receiving extra nutrients. All fruits and vegetables contain indigestible roughage which acts as an "intestinal broom" to keep the walls of your intestines from becoming clogged up with waste material. Folks who get a substantial portion of their calories from candy, soft drinks, white bread, cookies, and cake are cheating themselves of roughage which is needed to keep their intestinal tract in top condition (to say nothing of tooth decay and lost vitamins and minerals).

Dr. Clive M. McCay of Cornell, who is an authority on aging and nutrition, stated, "In no period of life is the proper functioning of the intestine more essential than in the later years." Dr. McCay found that the average length of life of a group of rats on a stock diet was 503 days. When he added 10 per cent more roughage to this diet, the average life increased to 674 days—a jump of 34 per cent!

AN APPROACH TO OPTIMAL CARBOHYDRATES

The recommendations from previous chapters indicate that we should get about 15 per cent of our calories from protein and about 25 per cent from fat. This leaves about 60 per cent of our calories from carbohydrates, for *there is no other source of calories.*

4. Stanley Davidson, A. P. Meiklejohn, R. Passmore, *Human Nutrition and Dietetics,* pp. 56-57. (Baltimore: The Williams and Wilkins Company, 1959.)

Carbohydrates from vegetables, fruits and grains should be used to fill the gap between our energy needs and the calories that are furnished by protein and fat.

But what are our calorie needs? This is a real problem, and you may not like the answer—I know I don't. Recent experiments by Dr. D. N. Berg have confirmed previous findings that fewer calories make for a longer life. They compared rats permitted to eat all they wanted with rats who were allowed to eat only about one-half as much. Those on half rations grew slowly and were slightly smaller in size. Dr. Berg found that sexual development was not retarded and degenerative diseases were delayed. The males on the low-calorie diet lived 25 per cent longer and the females lived 39 per cent longer! Even in old age, the low calorie animals ". . . resembled healthy young rats. Their fur was glossy, their teeth firm, and their activity lively." Although they were permitted fewer calories, they were well supplied with other nutrients. In contrast, the rats that could eat all the food they wanted ". . . became lethargic and had dull dirty fur and poor teeth." [5]

I regard this as very sad news indeed. It is too bad that such severe calorie restrictions seem to promote optimal health. Life insurance statistics loudly proclaim the health advantages of not loading yourself down with bulges of fat. The statistics clearly show that underweight folks live longer.

YOU'LL LIVE LONGER THINNER

World War II caused food restrictions in many European countries. In Sweden there was a decline in the rate of disease and death during the war years. When food became plentiful again after the war, the incidence of disease and death picked up. Do the stresses

5. *Nutrition Reviews*, Vol. 19, pp. 305-306, 1961.

of a world war cause tensions that affect the public health? Apparently we can stand up to stress pretty well if we avoid deficiencies and excesses in our nutrition. In Norway during the war, food supplies were low although there was no real famine. Before the war they had 91 deaths from tuberculosis per 100,000 people per year. The tuberculosis mortality figures steadily declined from 80 deaths per 100,000 in 1941 down to a low of 65 deaths per 100,000 in 1945. In countries where there was starvation and famine, the disease and death rate went up. But in countries where there was a *moderate reduction of the calorie supply*, better national health resulted.

Dr. Ancel Keys has pointed out that the typical American diet now has about 3,000 calories a day—and this is too much. He recommends that the level be lowered to 2,300 calories per day. This will result in a loss of weight for most people, but your weight will eventually become stabilized and you will probably benefit by less illness and greater longevity. The Vitamin-Mineral Index will help you make wise choices in reducing your calories.

"Half my friends have dug their graves with their teeth," said Chauncey Depew. Eating delicious foods is one of the ever-present dependable satisfactions that most of us enjoy three times a day. It seems a shame to recommend restraints on an activity that is so deeply satisfying. But sickness can limit happiness—and death can stop it completely. A wise person will not ignore the risks of obesity. An immature person usually grabs the pleasures he can today, and ignores the consequences of tomorrow. A mature person tries to achieve an intelligent balance between the present and the future. Only you can make the decision that will bring you the greatest total happiness over the rest of your life.

We thus find that there are two main things to

bear in mind in our approach to optimal carbohydrate intake. First, we should minimize refined carbohydrates such as sugar, candies, and soda pop, for these are lacking in vitamins and minerals that are needed by the body. Vegetables, fruits, grains, and milk are the best sources of carbohydrates. Second, if you are like most Americans, your problem is to cut down on the amount of carbohydrates you are getting in order to keep your weight within desirable limits. Chapter 2 gives additional information on achieving a desirable weight that will increase your life span. If you are careful about avoiding refined carbohydrates and keep your weight at a desirable level, you will probably be well on your way toward optimal carbohydrates. No further attention to carbohydrates seems to be necessary.

Chapter 9

THE VITAMIN–MINERAL INDEX

We were not designed to make our living sitting at desks or to spend our leisure hours slouched in a chair watching television while munching pretzels and sipping beer. Most of our ancestors, in order to survive in whatever degree of civilization they found themselves, had to live far more vigorous lives than we do. A man or woman living on a farm one hundred years ago may have used twice as much food as most Americans consume today. This probably provided them with far more calories, protein, vitamins and minerals than you and I obtain.

"Progress," said Bill Vaughn, "is a continuing effort to make the things we eat, drink and wear as good as they used to be." The Council on Foods and Nutrition of the American Medical Association has warned us of this trend toward "denatured" foods: "It is well known . . . that many foods have suffered deterioration in their nutritional values as a result of the influences of modern civilization. . . . The preference of the public for processed foods has frequently caused many of the valuable nutrients of a food to be discarded. . . . Examples of these effects may readily be found in the chemically pure sugar of commerce, which lacks all but traces of its original vitamins and minerals. . . . These 'denatured' foods have come to replace in large part the nutritious more nearly whole cereal grains which in former days supplied a considerable portion of the vitamins of the B group that enter the diet. . . . This is especially disturbing, since animal experiments have shown that ill effects resulting from less than satisfactory diets may become obvious only after many years." [1]

Many young children and teenagers today are being hurt through a lack of nutritional guidance and their reliance largely upon taste alone in making food choices. The clamor of soft drink ads and handy candy is overwhelming. I have seen even two-year-olds wheedle soft drinks and cookies from their mothers. Unfortunately these harassed mothers did not know that the 325 calories in one soft drink and two cookies were one-fourth of their child's daily calorie budget. These rather empty calories thus replaced more wholesome foods that their child needed for sturdy growth and good health.

The Council on Foods and Nutrition of the AMA deplores this unfortunate trend toward empty calories—especially with school children. "Empty calories" are calories that do not bear their fair share of the vitamins, minerals, protein, and unsaturated fats that your body needs for optimal health. The Council has recently stated, "The availability of confections and carbonated beverages on school premises may tempt children to spend lunch money for them and lead to poor food habits. Their high energy value and continual availability are likely to affect children's appetites for regular meals. Expenditures for carbonated beverages and most confections yield a nutritional return greatly inferior to that from milk, fruit, and other foods included in the basic food groups. When given a choice

1. Council on Foods and Nutrition, "Some Nutritional Aspects of Sugar, Candy and Sweetened Carbonated Beverages," *Journal of the American Medical Association*, Vol. 120, p. 763, 1942.

between carbonated beverages and milk or between candy and fruit, a child may choose the less nutritious. In view of these considerations, the Council on Foods and Nutrition is particularly opposed to the sale and distribution of confections and carbonated beverages in school lunchrooms."

THE VITAMIN-MINERAL INDEX

To help you deepen your knowledge of which foods make the highest contribution to your diet and which foods have calories that are largely "empty" of vitamins and minerals, I have devised a "Vitamin-Mineral Index." It is published for the first time in this book. You will find the Index in the Food Table.* The Vitamin-Mineral Index shows you the *average percentage of the daily allowance that is supplied by a 100-calorie portion of a food*. White potato, for example, has an Index of 8. This means that 100 calories of white potato can supply you with an average of 8 per cent of the daily recommended allowance for vitamins and minerals.

Here are the Vitamin-Mineral Indexes of some other foods:

Food	Index	Food	Index
Sugar	0	Cottage cheese	6
Hard candy	0	Whole milk	8
Soft drink	0	Wheat germ cereal	12
Jelly	1	Skim milk	14
Cookies	1	Oranges	27
Apple pie	1	Sweet potatoes	29
Corn flakes	2	Tomatoes	55
Pound cake	2	Beef liver	112
Sirloin steak	2	Carrots	148
Fresh pears	4	Mustard greens	212

* Page 214 explains the method used in computing the Vitamin-Mineral Index.

The Vitamin-Mineral Index is based on the *average* level of vitamins and minerals per calorie in each food. You will note, for example, that beef liver has a Vitamin-Mineral Index of 112. Sirloin steak only has an Index of 2. Although both meats are an excellent source of protein, liver has an average of about 56 times more vitamins and minerals per calorie! Use this handy guide to spot the foods that are high in vitamins and minerals.

If a particular food has a Vitamin-Mineral Index that is twice as high as another food, each calorie will contain double the average vitamin and mineral level of the other food. A high Index doesn't necessarily mean that a food is high in all vitamins and minerals. It means that *on the average*, it is high and can thus make a worthwhile contribution to your diet. The Index does not change with the quantity eaten—just as 100-octane gas remains 100-octane gas regardless of how much you use.

The Vitamin-Mineral Index is a wonderful tool to help you find the more nutritious foods. Like any tool, it can be misused. For example, it does not indicate the protein in a food, and so it is not fair to use the Index to compare beef with lettuce. Use it as a guide to *added nutritive values* when comparing meat with meat, cereal with cereal, vegetable with vegetable, and so forth. Always remember that your body needs protein and unsaturated fats as well as vitamins and minerals—and the Vitamin-Mineral Index only reflects the latter.

INCREASING NUTRITION DURING ILLNESS

Many of us fail to recognize that the less active we are, the more we should emphasize foods with high Vitamin-Mineral Indexes. For example, a person recuperating in bed needs fewer calories. His every mouthful should therefore be chosen from foods among those with more vitamins and minerals per calorie. But how many bedridden people, struggling for their health, understand this situation?

The Vitamin-Mineral Index can be a great boon to these people. If I were in bed fighting for my health, I would go through the Vitamin-Mineral Indexes in the Food Table and circle all the foods with the higher numbers. I would then work these unusually nutritious foods into my dietary pattern.

By using this convenient Index, you can quickly find the foods that will permit you to double your present vitamin and mineral intake and at the same time hold down your calories.

Folks in wheel chairs are also on limited-calorie budgets. If they wish to have the same vitamin and mineral intake as other members of the family (and to get it from wholesome foods rather than through pills), they will find this Vitamin-Mineral Index most helpful.

IF YOU'RE OVERWEIGHT

The Vitamin-Mineral Index can help you reduce your weight. The foods that have high Vitamin-Mineral Indexes have *very few calories in relation to their vitamins and minerals*. If you want to reduce, emphasize fruits and vegetables with Vitamin-Mineral Indexes over 25.

FOR ZEST IN OLD AGE

"Life doesn't begin at forty," said Red Skelton; "that's just when it begins to show." The Vitamin-Mineral Index can be helpful to older people who want the highest level of health. As people grow older, they need fewer calories. If they continue to eat the same amount of food as in their more active years, they will gain undesirable weight. If they cut down on their food without increasing the nutritional quality, they will have a lower vitamin and mineral intake. By choosing foods with higher Vitamin-Mineral Indexes, an elderly person can decrease his calories and at the same time have a vitamin and mineral level even higher than during youth!

DOGS HAVE IT BETTER

Some time ago I decided to find out if animal foods have more vitamins and minerals than those we eat. I wrote to the Ralston Purina Company, the world's largest feed manufacturer, and asked them to send me a laboratory analysis of their various animal foods. I was quite surprised when I computed the Vitamin-Mineral Indexes of foods *especially designed to keep animals in good health*. I found that their dog food has a Vitamin-Mineral Index of 30. Their laboratory feed for mice, rats, and hamsters has an Index of 38. Their monkey food has a Vitamin-Mineral Index of 22. The foods designed to maintain health in chicks, rabbits, foxes, and guinea pigs showed similarly high levels of vitamins and minerals. I then computed the Index of the diet recommended by the National Research Council for humans.* What a difference! I discovered that a diet meeting the recommended allowances of the National Research Council only has an average Vitamin-Mineral Index of 3! This was most shocking.

Why this enormous difference between animal and

---

* These computations of the Vitamin-Mineral Index are based on the procedure given on page 214 of this book. A 3,200-calorie diet that meets the allowance for the reference man was used as a basis for computing the Vitamin-Mineral Index of a diet recommended by the National Research Council. Since numerous animals make their own vitamin C and thus do not require a dietary source, this vitamin was omitted from the computation. The Vitamin-Mineral Index for food designed for these animals is based on the remaining five nutrients.

human food? Why do the foods designed to keep animals in good health have *many times* more vitamins and minerals per calorie than the National Research Council recommends for humans? Could it be that animals need far more vitamins and minerals per calorie than you and I? Probably not. Are our excessive illnesses and high medical, surgical, and hospital bills associated with the low vitamin-mineral values of the foods some people select? Evidence to give final answers to these questions is not yet available, but I, for one, resolved to gradually modify my own diet so that the Vitamin-Mineral Indexes of most of my foods are as good as those used to keep dogs, rats, and monkeys in good health. If you want to join me in this adventure in nutritious eating, let the Food Table be your guide.

HOW DO YOU REACT TO NEW FOODS?

To some extent, animals and even very young children have an "instinct" for making wise food choices. You and I lack this. We are governed by taste and habit and these can lead us far astray. If you want to take advantage of some of the foods with higher Vitamin-Mineral Indexes, you may need to get acquainted with foods you haven't used before. Some people like to try new foods; some would rather die first. Many intelligent folks realize that *taste preferences are largely childhood habits.* Psychologist Kurt Lewin said that we don't just eat the foods we like— we tend to like the foods we eat!

Most people find that by nibbling a food that is new to them, they will probably in time broaden their taste to include it. Did you like your first olive? When you are aware of the nutritional contribution a food can make in your journey toward optimal nutrition, your intelligence may help you gradually work it into your food pattern.

Chapter 10

LET'S BE GENEROUS WITH VITAMIN A

When a man with night blindness went to see Hippocrates, the ancient Greek father of medicine, he was instructed to "eat, once or twice, as big an ox liver as possible, raw, and dipped in honey." After nearly 2,300 years, this sugar-coated prescription is still an excellent one—although we now know how to get the same benefit in a more palatable way.

If you are deficient in vitamin A, your eyes will become increasingly affected by glare at night. Bright headlights of oncoming cars will have an uncomfortable blinding effect. You probably think this is normal and blame it on the car designers in Detroit. If vitamin A is scarce, you may have difficulty adjusting your sight when you go from bright daylight to find a seat in a dark theater. If it takes you several minutes to see what you're doing, the chances are pretty good that you are deficient in vitamin A.

One of the functions of vitamin A in your body is to make a substance called "visual purple," which is used in the retina of your eye to increase your ability to see in dim light. Bright glaring lights use it up rapidly. If adequate vitamin A is available, it is replaced almost instantaneously. If you're low in vitamin A, it is replaced slowly and in the meantime your vision is impaired.

Drivers who are very deficient in vitamin A can barely see a few feet ahead at night. Their failure to see road signs has caused many accidents. Many people suffer from eyestrain when watching television. They have been surprised by their freedom from eyestrain after they improved their nutrition. Some folks low in vitamin A wear dark glasses at night in an unknowing attempt to protect their small supply of "visual purple" made from vitamin A. When a person low in vitamin A moves to a new job where the room is brightly illuminated, he may develop severe eyestrain. A better diet would avoid this problem, one that could make him give up his job.

A VITAMIN OF MANY FUNCTIONS

Vitamin A is vital to life. If it is supplied in meager amounts, growth will be retarded. Vitamin A profoundly affects development of the teeth. When tooth buds buried in a child's jaw are ready to receive a hard coat of enamel to protect them over the years, the enamel-forming cells will not do their job well if vitamin A is undersupplied. The enamel will be pockmarked with tiny pits. These may later catch food deposits, which will ferment and form acids that eat away enamel and leave decay.[1] A soft lovely skin cannot be maintained without this vitamin. It is helpful in developing soft lustrous hair and attractive fingernails.

Experiments have shown that a lack of vitamin A may severely influence reproduction. Male rats on vita-

1. Ernestine B. McCollum and Elmer V. McCollum, "Vitamins A, D, E, K," from *Food, The Yearbook of Agriculture 1959*, Department of Agriculture, p. 131. (Washington, D.C.: U.S. Government Printing Office.)

min A deficient diets were unable to make sperm, and females lacking in this vitamin were unable to bear young.[2]

This vitamin is essential to help you maintain a strong first line of defense against certain types of infection. Many of the organs of your body are lined with specialized cells which secrete a protective coat of mucous. This thin, sticky fluid acts as a trap for invading bacteria. When you have a cold, the cells in your nasal passages are particularly active in producing large amounts of mucous to trap the invading germs before they have an opportunity to penetrate into your tissues.

Tissues at body openings that come in contact with bacilli from the outside world are provided with this protective mucous barrier. These include the nasal and throat passages, lungs, uterus, vagina, and the urinary tract. If you have been low in vitamin A, the cells lining these organs will tend to dry up, flatten, and slough off and no longer provide the tissues with protective secretions. In addition, tiny hairlike cilia that keep the surface clean by constant movement will disappear. This leaves the door wide open to trouble. Severe infections of your eyes, mouth, lungs, genitals, or urinary tracts may result. Vitamin A will not keep you from getting colds, but an adequate supply may keep your cold from progressing to more serious things by maintaining your body defenses against invading bacteria. When investigators injected infections into groups of animals, the ones liberally supplied with vitamin A fought the infection more effectively and did not become so ill.

It is important when reading a book on nutrition to be cautious in using a reverse type of reasoning. For

2. George D. Wolf, *Nutrition Reviews*, Vol. 20, No. 6, p. 163, June, 1962.

example, when you read that lack of vitamin A retards growth, it does not necessarily follow that a child who has failed to grow is lacking in vitamin A. *Most bodily symptoms can be produced by a host of different causes.*

WHERE TO GET IT

The livers of all animals are excellent sources of vitamin A. The liver, as the chemical workshop of the body, stores this vitamin, as well as other vitamins and minerals. You will note, for example, in the Food Table that three ounces of beef liver will provide 910 per cent of your recommended daily allowance of vitamin A. It has over nine hundred times more vitamin A than sirloin steak! Lamb liver, beef liver, chicken liver, calf liver and pork liver are all excellent sources. If pork liver is used, be sure to cook it well to kill any lurking organisms. The older the animal, the more vitamin A will be stored in the liver.

Fish-liver oils are rich in vitamin A. Small shellfish eat the green plant algae of the ocean and they are eaten by larger fish which are, in turn, eaten by still bigger fish until we find large concentrations of vitamin A developing in the liver of fish such as the cod and halibut. Cod-liver oil has long been famous for its health-giving supply of vitamins A and D, to say nothing of its rather fishy smell. The liver of the percomorph fishes, such as halibut, yields such a concentration of vitamin A that a few drops of oleum percomorphum will do the job of a teaspoon of cod-liver oil.

Vitamin A, as such, occurs only in animal foods. Plants contain beta carotene, which your body can convert into vitamin A. Green foods, such as turnip greens and broccoli, have large amounts of carotene which give them unusually high vitamin A values. The figures shown in our Food Table represent vitamin A values which include a proper allowance for your body's ability to convert carotene to vitamin A.

Vitamin A values occur in the greatest amounts in yellow-colored vegetables such as carrots and sweet potatoes and in plants with thin green leaves such as turnip greens, mustard greens, kale, etc. You will note that a half-cup of cooked carrots provides 181 per cent of your daily vitamin A allowance. As you have probably noticed in the Food Table, other foods rich in vitamin A values include apricots, broccoli, pumpkin, cantaloupe, and tomatoes. The yellower the turnips and peaches, the higher the vitamin A value.

A quarter-pound stick of butter contains 75 per cent of the daily vitamin A allowance. Margarine is now usually enriched by the addition of a similar amount of vitamin A. Both butter and margarine, however, contain saturated fat which must be used sparingly if you are not to exceed the suggested levels of fat outlined in Chapter 7.

Skim milk in which the butterfat has been removed is now being fortified with vitamin A. In some areas, skim milk is available with both vitamin A and D added. A quart of this milk contains 40 per cent of your daily allowance for vitamin A plus an adequate supply of vitamin D. It is more economical than whole milk and is extremely helpful to anyone who wants to have the benefits of a quart or more of milk per day without running up his saturated fat total.

CHOOSE QUALITY FRUITS AND VEGETABLES

A word of caution is needed. Although the Food Table says that a half-cup of carrots supplies 181 per cent of your daily allowance for vitamin A, it is important to remember that it isn't necessarily so. The nutrient values given in the Food Table are *average* values. A half-cup of light-colored carrots may have only 50 per cent of the daily vitamin A allowance. Others with a deep rich orange color have two and one-half times the value shown in the Table!

Dr. Sherman has emphasized that full vitamin A values can be expected only in leaves that are fully green. He warns us, "Leaves which are relatively colorless must be expected to be of low vitamin A value. Thus Kramer and co-workers found less than one-thirtieth as much vitamin A value in the white inner leaves of head lettuce as in the green outer leaves of the same plants. And the white inner leaves of tight-headed cabbages are of very much less vitamin A value than the green leaves of the loose-leaf cabbages. . . ." [3]

If a vegetable is rubbery, don't buy it. A tired vegetable, which may have lost some of its vitamins, will not meet the standards of our Food Table. Diseased, malnourished plants that did not grow vigorously should never find their way to market. Unfortunately, some housewives' standards for vegetables are so low that these inferior quality plants are frequently purchased. "They are going to be cooked anyhow," a housewife may say, "so what difference does it make?" If you are content with lifeless greens, anemic carrots, and pale sweet potatoes, you may be fooling yourself when you use the values in the Food Table.

PROTECTION FROM LOSS

It has been found that an adequate supply of vitamin E will help to stretch your supply of vitamin A. Vitamin C has also been found to help preserve vitamin A inside your body. Your program of optimal nutrition should enable you to store a two- to three-year supply of vitamin A in your liver.

For years physicians have cautioned us against the use of mineral oil. When it is present in the intestines, it will grab and hold the oil-soluble vitamins. Since mineral oil is not a food, it cannot be used by the body. The oil-soluble vitamins will ultimately be lost to you when your body gets rid of the mineral oil.

Vitamin A is not easily destroyed by ordinary methods of cooking. However, it is destroyed by rancidity. Any food that smells even slightly rancid should be chucked in the garbage can, since it can be irritating to the stomach and intestines. Vitamin A can also be damaged in fruits that are dried at high temperatures or in the sun. Sulphur-dried apricots are protected against this loss.

The loss of vitamins is generally retarded by storage of foods in a cool, dark place. Since the purpose of your refrigerator is to preserve taste and nutritive values, it is best to store vegetables there. Unlike some vitamins, vitamin A stores well in cans. Cooked carrots sealed in airtight containers in 1824 for the Arctic voyage of the H. M. S. *Hecla* were discovered in 1939. When opened and analyzed, they had approximately the same vitamin A value as a fresh carrot.[4]

Humans do not have enzymes that can break down the cellulose wall that encloses all plant cells. The more thoroughly you chew a raw vegetable, the more these fiber walls will be broken down by grinding between your molars. Cooking ruptures these cell walls to make the oil-soluble vitamins more available. Dr. Elmer V. McCollum, the co-discoverer of vitamin A, has pointed

---

4. Stanley Davidson, A. P. Meiklejohn, R. Passmore, *Human Nutrition and Dietetics,* p. 204. (Baltimore: The William and Wilkins Company, 1959.)

out that when cooked carrots are put through a blender, vitamin A availability is doubled as compared with cooked carrots, whether sliced or mashed. Puréeing of this type may be helpful to infants or young children or elderly folks without teeth.

Vitamin A dissolves in oil but not in water. When liver is eaten, there is enough fat or oil in it to carry vitamin A into your blood. Since vegetables such as greens or carrots are almost fat-free, you get the greatest benefit from their vitamin A value when they are eaten with a meal containing a small amount of fat. Bile produced by the liver is also needed for the proper absorption of vitamin A and other fat soluble vitamins. People with colitis or obstruction of the bile ducts may not be able to absorb these vitamins. For these folks, physicians will freqeuntly recommend vitamin A acetate capsules which do not have to combine with fat to enter the blood.[5]

INADVISABLE IN HUGE AMOUNTS

Eskimo and Arctic explorers have learned to stay away from polar-bear liver. Two groups of explorers had to learn this the hard way. Both expeditions reported loss of skin from head to foot of men who ate polar-bear liver. An analysis of this liver showed that someone eating only three and one-half ounces of polar bear liver would get about four hundred times the recommended daily allowance of vitamin A!

Dr. A. Gerber reported the unusual case of a 21-year-old woman who maintained a daily intake of one hundred times the recommended allowance for vitamin A to treat a skin condition.[6] She continued this

5. B. M. Kagan, "Vitamin A," from Michael G. Wohl, Robert S. Goodhart, eds., *Modern Nutrition in Health and Disease*, 2nd ed., pp. 292-293. (Philadelphia: Lea and Febiger, 1960.)

6. A. Gerber, A. P. Raab, and A. E. Sobel, *American Journal of Medicine*, Vol. 16, p. 729, 1954.

over a nine-year period and was in and out of six hospitals. Symptoms began with headaches, double vision, and nausea. In the first hospital she received a tentative diagnosis of brain tumor, and throughout a long comedy of errors (it wasn't funny to her) she accumulated about a dozen diagnoses, including serous meningitis, chronic encephalitis, Addison's disease, and infectious hepatitis. She underwent several operations. Having received no help in hospitals, she turned to chiropractors and osteopaths, but without improvement. During all this time she continued faithfully to take vitamin A capsules that were providing her with one hundred times the recommended allowance each day!

After eight years, with things getting worse all the time, she finally went to a hospital where a nutrition-conscious doctor associated her terribly high intake of vitamin A with her long string of difficulties. A test showed that she had the highest vitamin A concentration ever found in human blood. The self-administered vitamin A capsules were immediately stopped and she was put on a normal diet. At the end of one month her skin texture improved and her bone pains were markedly diminished. Two months after vitamin A had been discontinued, all spontaneous pain had gone and she continued to gain weight and improve steadily until signs of vitamin A poisoning vanished.

Some mothers accustomed to giving cod-liver oil by the spoonful have not realized that highly concentrated *percomorph oil should be given in drops*. Cases have been recorded in which infants and young children have for several months received twenty to one hundred times the recommended adult allowance for vitamin A. The AMA Council on Foods and Nutrition does not approve of any capsule that provides more than five times the recommended daily allowance for vitamin A.

From the above it should be obvious that vitamin A poisoning requires enormously large dosages of pills or fish-liver oils. Vitamin A poisoning is no problem to one eating a diet of natural foods available in the United States. Let us therefore leave this subject of vitamin A overdosage to those who think that if one capsule is good, ten will be better.

WORKING TOWARD OPTIMAL VITAMIN A

You will note that the Food Table shows the percentage of the recommended allowance for vitamin A for all listed foods. *If the foods you eat during a day add up to a vitamin A score of 100 per cent, you will be receiving the recommended allowance of the National Research Council for adult men and women.* This is about 50 per cent more than the minimum needed to avoid deficiency symptoms. You will note in the table entitled "Recommended Allowances for Various Groups" on page 216 that the vitamin A allowance for women in the second half of pregnancy should total 120 per cent. It should go to 160 per cent while nursing. Pediatricians usually prescribe suitable amounts for infants under one year. From one to three years, a child should have a vitamin A total of 40 per cent. This should be increased steadily as shown on the table on page 216 as the child grows.

As you will recall from Chapter 1, Sherman found that Diet A was adequate and permitted over seventy generations of laboratory animals to thrive. However, when vitamin A was quadrupled with no other change in the diet, the males lived 10.4 per cent longer and the females 12.1 per cent longer. The prime of life between the attainment of maturity and the onset of old age *was increased by an even greater percentage.* He found that the optimal intake of vitamin A was at least four times and not more than eight times the minimal-adequate level.[7]

It has been found that when your body has been generously supplied with vitamin A above the recommended level, more of the vitamin will be used by your tissues. Since lifetime experiments have never been made with human beings, no one knows for sure where the human optimal level should be placed. The evidence from animal experiments, however, appears to indicate overwhelmingly that you will benefit by a generous daily intake. Sherman's experiments with Diet A led him to state, "There is no doubt that in these experiments the addition of extra vitamin A to a diet which already contained 'enough of everything' did positively and constructively build higher health and longer life. And we need have no doubt that this same thing may often occur with people." [8]

You, as an individual, may require a larger or smaller amount of vitamin A than average. In order to allow for individual variation, and to enable you to build a large reserve of this vitamin, it may be beneficial to select foods so that your vitamin A total each day comes to at least 250 per cent. By the generous use of liver and green vegetables in my own diet, I frequently have a daily vitamin A total of 500 per cent. I'm not going to let Sherman's rats get ahead of me!

7. Henry C. Sherman, *The Nutritional Improvement of Life*, p. 184. (New York: Columbia University Press, 1950.)
8. Henry C. Sherman, *op. cit.*, p. 467.

Chapter 11

BENEFICIAL B VITAMINS

"I certainly hope I'm sick," said the unhappy man to his doctor. "I'd sure hate to feel like this if I'm well." A shortage of B vitamins could be responsible for this below-par feeling. There are at least twelve B vitamins that have so far been discovered, and research is hot on the trail of additional ones. In this chapter we will get acquainted with vitamins B_1 and B_2, which are included in our Food Table, and then briefly touch upon the others.

You will recall that vitamin A is oil soluble and needs fat or oil to carry it into the blood stream. The term "B-complex" refers to the large group of *water*-soluble vitamins listed in this chapter. In the next chapter we will discuss the best sources of the B-complex vitamins and also show you how you can work toward optimal levels of these vitamins without complicating your Nutrition Analysis.

VITAMIN B_1 (THIAMINE)

Millions of people have died because of a lack of B_1. Nature provided each grain of rice with a hull in which B-complex vitamins are concentrated. Man learned to remove the hull and to value only the white portion that is so low in vitamins and minerals. Countless deaths in the Orient have resulted from this nutritional sabotage.

Around 1880 there were about 5,000 enlisted men in the Japanese Navy. Each year beriberi hit from 20 to 40 per cent of the entire fleet. Dr. Takaki, a Navy medical officer, got permission to make a nutritional experiment. A warship with 276 men aboard was sent on a nine-month cruise from Japan to New Zealand, Chile, Honolulu, and back. The diet consisted largely of white rice. During this time there were 169 cases of beriberi with 25 deaths. On a similar vessel making the same journey, the rice was decreased and more barley plus vegetables, meat, and condensed milk were added to the sailors' diet. On this cruise covering the same time and the same ports, only 14 men contracted beriberi—and each of these had failed to eat his share of the new foods. After Dr. Takaki's convincing demonstration, the entire Japanese Navy used less white rice. Soon there were practically no cases of this often fatal disease.

Subsequent work around 1900 revealed that beriberi was due to a lack of B_1—the first B vitamin to be discovered. It was later named "thiamine." When starches and sugars are converted into energy for the cells, pyruvic acid accumulates as a waste product. If B_1 is not adequately supplied, your blood will bog down with chemical garbage and you are on the sick list.

THE MORALE VITAMIN

Dr. R. D. Williams designed an experiment to find out the effects of a shortage of B_1.[1] His subject, whom we will call Betty, was given a good start with a large amount of B_1. After this saturation dose, each day Betty received 71 per cent of the recommended allowance of the National Research Council. During this period her health was excellent, and the scientists working with her considered her congenial, industrious, efficient, and vigorous.

Then her intake of B_1 was dropped to about 40 per cent of the recommended allowance. At the end of two months, the investigators noted that Betty worked slowly, often neglected her work, followed instructions inaccurately, was forgetful, irritable, quarrelsome, and had a capricious appetite. Her basal metabolism dropped considerably and her energy level was low. During the next two months, Betty had the same B_1-deficient diet and her symptoms grew worse. At times she would be found weeping and then she would break out laughing. She became very critical of herself and worked irregularly. She was apathetic, confused, fatigued, and had numbness of hands and feet in addition to frequent nausea and pain.

As she continued on the diet that provided only 40 per cent of her recommended allowance, Betty really broke down. She often was unable to work because of dizziness and weakness. She had a hopeless attitude and was confused and bewildered. At times she was apathetic, then agitated. She was depressed and had pallor

1. R. D. Williams, H. L. Mason, B. F. Smith, and R. M. Wilder, "Induced Thiamine (Vitamin B_1) Deficiency and the Thiamine Requirement of Man; Further Observations," *Archives of Internal Medicine*, Vol. 69, p. 721, 1942.

and giddiness when standing. Her hands and feet were cold and mottled and her heart beat irregularly. After approximately six months, the scientists began to add small amounts of B_1 to Betty's diet. Very little improvement was noticed for six weeks. When more was added to her diet she gradually improved, but tired easily and slept poorly. When Betty's intake of B_1 was increased to meet the allowance of the National Research Council, all symptoms disappeared.

The troubles experienced by this anonymous heroine of nutritional research have also been duplicated in other experiments involving larger numbers of men and women. Vitamin B_1 has been called the "morale vitamin," for a shortage may result in irritability, forgetfulness, confusion, and fear. Other scientists have found that a deficiency in vitamin B_1 resulted in loss of emotional control, manic-depressive behavior, suspicion of persecution, sensitivity to pain, general weakness, and extreme lack of appetite.

While most nutritional deficiencies gradually reduce your appetite, a lack of B_1 will cause it to lag more quickly than a deficiency of any other vitamin. B_1 also restores your appetite more quickly than any other known nutrient. Many mothers for whom mealtime is an unhappy bite-by-bite struggle may make life more beautiful for themselves and their children if they serve more foods rich in B_1.

Vitamin B_1 is known to stimulate the strong rhythmic contraction of the intestines needed to rid the body of food waste. The emptying time of the intestines and stomach has been found to be nearly twice as slow in B_1-deficient animals as in normal ones. This vitamin has been helpful in relieving stubborn cases of constipation.

B_1 is not stored well in the body, and your limited supply is readily exhausted by fever, surgical operations,

or other stresses. As shown in the "Recommended
Allowances for Various Groups" on page 216, pregnant and nursing women need to boost their B₁ total.

SOURCES OF B₁

Dr. Margaret Chaney has observed, "There is a
trend toward low levels of thiamine [B₁] in the diet." [2]
You have probably noticed in the Food Table that most
foods contain very little B₁. The best sources for vitamin
B₁ are organ meats such as heart, kidney, and liver, and
wheat germ, yeast, rice bran or rice polish, lean pork,
and soybeans. As much as one-third of the B₁ in foods
may be destroyed by boiling, but practically none is lost
when the vegetables are steamed.

VITAMIN B₂ (RIBOFLAVIN)

By reading about each vitamin separately, you
might get the idea that each works independently of
others in the body. Nothing could be further from the
truth. Most vitamins combine with other vitamins, minerals, and protein to make enzymes and coenzymes,
which interact with each other and affect every cell in
the body. The B-complex vitamins are particularly
interwoven into the process of converting food into
energy. Sugar alone is of no use to your cells unless
accompanied by various B vitamins. These vitamins are
needed as the sugar reaches the cells and after it is used
by them, to remove waste products.

It is possible that you may have occasionally
noticed symptoms that could have been due to a shortage of B₂ in your body. A lack of B₂ may cause your

2. Margaret S. Chaney, *Nutrition*, 6th ed., p. 277. (Boston:
The Riverside Press, 1960.)

lips to become sore, dry, and chapped; they may split open at the ends. These painful cracks at the corners of the mouth usually do not bleed but do not heal readily. A long-standing deficiency of vitamin B_2 may cause little wrinkles to radiate out from the mouth—as when you pucker your lips or whistle.

The whites of your eyes are made up of tissue that is remarkable for its ability to survive without a circulating blood supply in the immediate vicinity. The tears that bathe your eye contain considerable amounts of vitamin B_2. When undersupplied, it may be necessary for the whites of your eyes to grow small blood vessels. This gives you a "hungover" bloodshot appearance which will probably disappear in a few weeks if vitamin B_2 is adequately supplied. A lack of vitamin A can also result in plugging up your tear ducts and giving you bloodshot eyes.

Sunglasses might be far less popular if people had adequate supplies of vitamin B_2. A deficiency of this vitamin will make your eyes hurt from what you think is too much glaring light *in the daytime*. Bill S. was careful to wear sunglasses whenever he went boating or swimming. Bright sidewalks in the sunshine bothered his eyes. White clouds and light skies made him squint. After I helped him develop a program of optimal nutrition, he suddenly realized one day that a month had passed in which he had forgotten to put on his dark glasses! His generous supply of vitamin B_2 did the trick.

You will recall from the last chapter that a lack of vitamin A will dim your night vision and make your eyes painfully sensitive to glare *at night*. Stinginess with vitamin B_2 can give you teary, burning eyes, dim your vision, and eventually, if the deficiency continues, your eyes may become opaque and your vision is lost. When it comes to vitamins A and B₂, make sure the "eyes have it."

The *Journal of the American Medical Association* has called vitamin B₂ "essential to the defense powers of the organism." A generous intake of B₂ makes a marked difference when experimental animals are exposed to certain infections. When virulent bacilli are injected into animals, the survival and recovery rate is higher if they are well supplied with this vitamin. A deficiency in B₂ may cause a severe breaking out on the scrotum of men and the vagina of women. Shortage of B₂ can often bring about changes in the tongue. In addition to soreness and burning, it may turn purplish-red or magenta. The taste buds can atrophy so that much of the taste of food is lost. Highly seasoned foods may be irritating.

Dr. V. P. Sydenstricker considered a deficiency of B₂ to be the most common vitamin deficiency in the United States. Liver and kidneys, wheat germ, yeast, eggs, milk, and milk products are the richest source of this vitamin.

BUILDING A HIGHER LEVEL OF HEALTH

The most wonderful thing about vitamin B₂ lies not in the diseases it prevents, but in its ability to build a higher level of health. When optimally supplied, vitamin B₂ (riboflavin) probably shares with vitamin A and calcium the ability to help you increase your resistance to disease and add to your prime of life and longevity. Dr. Henry Sherman found that a generous supply above the adequate level ". . . tends to result in better development, higher adult vitality, greater freedom from disease at all ages, somewhat longer life, and (more significantly) a longer 'prime of life,' i.e., a longer segment of the life cycle between the attainment of adult capacity and the onset of old age." [3]

"Recommended Allowances for Various Groups" on page 216 shows that women in the second half of pregnancy should have a B_2 score of 111 per cent. This should be run up to 139 per cent while nursing. The needs of teenage boys and girls are also high. In referring to the National Research Council's recommended allowances for B_2, Sherman states, ". . . All the experiments with human beings have been for too short periods to show what the allowance would need to be to bring optimal well-being (so far as this factor is concerned) throughout the normal life cycle. The present Recommended Allowances are, in the judgment of the present writer, more than minimal adequate but less than fully optimal." [4]

NIACIN

Niacin is a B-complex vitamin, but it is known by a name rather than a number. It is important to remember that most of the B vitamins are concerned with releasing the energy in food. This means that they play vital roles in the incredibly complex and incompletely understood chemical processes which must take place when you convert food into energy. When wood is burned, it creates energy by producing heat. When food is "burned" in the body, it must take place at body temperature. Perhaps nowhere else in nature is this miracle of low-temperature burning of fuel accomplished outside of living organisms. If you have a shortage of B vitamins, some of the links in the chain of energy production will be impaired. In the description

3. Reprinted with permission of The Macmillan Company from *Chemistry of Food and Nutrition* by Henry C. Sherman. Eighth edition Copyright 1952 by The Macmillan Company.
4. *Ibid.*, p. 404.

of the remaining B vitamins that follows, you will notice that many of them have similar symptoms when they are insufficiently supplied. A deficiency in only one of the B vitamins is not likely. A diet that is low in one of them will most likely be low in several or in all.

For many years, some folks in rural areas in the South who lived on a diet of corn meal, fatty salt pork, dried beans, and molasses were plagued with pellagra. This became known as the disease of the four D's— dermatitis, diarrhea, dementia, and death. In 1935, Dr. Tom Spies reported that he had been able to reduce the mortality rate in severe pellagra from 54 per cent to 6 per cent. He did this by giving yeast or liver extracts and by making sure in every case that the patient ate a diet high in calories, protein, minerals, and vitamins. He found that a daily intake of four ounces of wheat germ, two ounces of yeast, or two ounces of liver extract would prevent pellagra. Before the discovery of the B vitamin niacin, the campaign to stamp out this often fatal disease emphasized the use of protein foods and leafy vegetables.

The National Research Council has made recommendations for the daily intake of niacin, but no food tables for niacin values are available covering a large variety of foods. Data is available showing the *amount* of niacin in the foods of our table, but this does not tell the whole story because your body can make this vitamin if well supplied with tryptophane, an essential amino acid available in any complete protein. The richest sources of niacin materials are liver and other organ meats, wheat germ, yeast, rice bran or rice polish, peanuts, and tuna fish.

VITAMIN B$_6$ (PYRIDOXINE)

Most of the B vitamins act as links in a chain. When the B$_6$ link is broken, we get many effects that are similar to those observed when the B$_1$, B$_2$, or niacin links are broken. Research has shown that a deficiency in vitamin B$_6$ may result in lack of appetite, nausea, lethargy, breaking out of the skin, and cracks in the corners of the lips. It has also been found to slow down the production of antibodies which your body needs to increase your resistance to disease. Deposits of cholesterol in the arteries of monkeys increased when there was a deficiency of this vitamin.

When vitamin B$_6$ is undersupplied, there is a growth failure in infants and a severe skin rash may break out. A few years ago the heat used in sterilizing a certain baby food destroyed the B$_6$ it contained. Infants throughout the nation using this food developed irritability, muscular twitchings, and convulsive seizures. This was corrected quickly when the error in processing was discovered.

Dr. Tom Spies found that a deficiency in this vitamin was associated with weakness, nervousness, insomnia, irritability, abdominal pain, and difficulty in walking. He found that these symptoms disappeared when he prescribed vitamin B$_6$. There appears to be an increased need for this vitamin by older folks.

It has been found that when meat is roasted or stewed, from 20 to 50 per cent of this vitamin may be lost. Yeast, liver and other organ meats, wheat germ, and rice bran or rice polish are among the richest sources.

PANTOTHENIC ACID

The queen bee lives for about five years while the worker bees live only one summer. This difference in longevity seems to have a nutritional basis. The larvae that are fed "royal jelly" develop into queen bees. Experiments have shown that pantothenic acid in royal jelly is responsible for this great increase in longevity. These facts led the fast-buck boys to sell royal jelly with claims of adding longevity, restoring potency, rejuvenating sagging breasts, correcting gray hair, and a myriad of other fantastic claims, until the Food and Drug Administration hauled them into court. In spite of the fact that it does not work miracles, pantothenic acid has an important part to play in human nutrition.

During the war many American prisoners on poor diets developed a painful "burning" sensation in their feet. Numbness and tingling of the toes was followed by burning and shooting pains. Vitamins B_1, B_2, and niacin did not help, but pantothenic acid brought relief.

Pantothenic acid has been called the "antistress vitamin." Experiments with humans deficient in pantothenic acid resulted in weakness, fatigue, decrease in spontaneous activity, changes in mood, psychosis, dizziness, unsteadiness in walking, cramps, and torpor. It has been found to help in reducing cramps in pregnant women. This vitamin is widely distributed among foods. The richest sources are organ meats, yeast, wheat germ, and rice bran or rice polish.

VITAMIN B_{12} (CYANOCOBALAMIN)

In the past, pernicious anemia was a disease as dreaded as advanced cancer; it was invariably fatal. But in 1926, Minot and Murphy saved lives by advising patients to eat seven ounces of liver daily—á la Hippocrates. When B_{12} was isolated in 1948, it was found that as little as one-millionth of a gram injected per day can change a person dying with pernicious anemia into a well person. (A gram is about one-twenty-eighth of an ounce.) People with pernicious anemia have a disorder in their gastric secretions that prevents the absorption of this vitamin.

B_{12} is known to be made by bacilli in the intestines, but it is uncertain how much of this is available for absorption. The nerves of the central nervous system seem to be dependent on it. Unlike the other B vitamins, it stores well in the liver, and a B_{12}-rich diet may permit a three-year supply to be stockpiled. Pregnancy increases the need for this vitamin.

Liver and kidney are the best sources of vitamin B_{12}. Some Torula yeasts contain about a day's supply per half ounce. Vegetarian diets are usually lacking in adequate B_{12}, for only insignificant traces are found in fruits, vegetables, and grains. It has been found, for example, that even a confirmed vegetarian such as the guinea pig will grow better when small amounts of B_{12}-rich meats are included in his diet.

BIOTIN

Biotin deficiency in man results in changes in the skin and tongue, loss of appetite, heart symptoms, lassitude, and intense depression with hallucinations. Much experimental work remains to be done on biotin as well as many of the other lesser-known B vitamins. Their roles in the chemistry of the body are poorly understood. Like ships that pass in the night, we don't know yet exactly where they've been or where they're going.

Avidin, a substance in raw egg white, will combine with biotin and make it unavailable to your body

Cooking an egg prevents this. One man whose habitual diet consisted of ten raw eggs daily washed down by a pint of red wine suffered from severe dermatitis and eye trouble. This cleared up when the raw eggs were stopped and biotin was supplied along with a normal diet. Many babies fed a formula with raw eggs have broken out with painful skin rashes that disappear when the raw egg white is omitted.

OTHER B VITAMINS

Folic acid, another B vitamin, has been found to be effective in curing certain types of anemia, but it does not help anemia when due to lack of iron. It will alleviate some of the symptoms of pernicious anemia but cannot stop the fatal course of this disease. This led the AMA Council on Foods and Drugs to suggest that the folic acid in vitamin preparations be held to a minimum to avoid hiding the symptoms of pernicious anemia. Folic acid plays an important part in the creation of new cells.

Inositol, choline, and para-aminobenzoic acid are also B vitamins about which too little is known. They are supplied by the same foods that are the best sources of the other B vitamins.

THE B COMPLEX AND YOUR HEALTH

The importance of vitamins in maintaining a high level of health that will raise your body's defense against disease was demonstrated in an experiment by Dr. F. E. Tisdall of the University of Toronto. He compared the infection-survival rates of different groups of rats that were deficient in A, D, and the B vitamins. He injected them with an active bacillus and found that only 40 per cent of the A-deficient rats survived as compared to 79 per cent of the rats on an adequate diet. He found that 28 per cent of the D-deficient rats survived as compared to 55 per cent of the well-fed ones. Those deficient in B vitamins fared worst of all. Only 20 per cent of this group survived the infection as compared with 72 per cent of those receiving a generous supply of the B complex.

Sometimes surprising things happen when your body is treated to generous quantities of the B complex for several months. One man I know whose diet appeared to meet the recommended allowances of the National Research Council found a remarkable increase in sex interest and ability after he began taking two ounces of yeast daily. From once or twice a week, he began to gradually achieve a daily sex pattern. His many evidences of increased health, including added virility, have thus far been sustained for a three-year period since he began using two ounces of yeast per day *in addition to making his diet as optimal as he could in other ways.*

In considering the matter of increased sex interest, it is important to emphasize but not to overemphasize the importance of the B complex. Basically sex is a function of health. Anything that adds to your health probably adds to this vital aspect of your life. Although B vitamins can produce a remarkable increase in vitality and joy of living, they cannot do the job alone. Your highest physical peak can only be attained when you also work toward optimal amounts of other vitamins, minerals, protein, fat, and carbohydrate.

Chapter 12

THE ROAD TO OPTIMAL B VITAMINS

"Optimum nutrition," said Dr. D. Mark Hegsted of Harvard, "is somewhere in between too little and too much; and the definition of it really is our major problem in nutrition." [1] The pinpointing of optimal amounts of the B-complex vitamins at this time is impossible. Even recommended allowances are not available from the National Research Council for most of these vitamins.

The various B vitamins are widely distributed throughout many foods. Meats, milk, eggs, peas and beans, green vegetables, and whole grain breads and cereals are among the better sources of a few of these vitamins. *However, none of these foods supply excellent amounts of the entire B complex.*

Fortunately, there is an intelligent program you can follow which will probably help you get nearly optimal amounts of the B complex. Dr. L. Jean Bogert in her book *Nutrition and Physical Fitness* suggests liver, wheat germ, yeast, and bran as excellent foods that offer larger amounts of the B vitamins. Dr. Bogert

1. D. Mark Hegsted, "Some Consequences of Overnutrition with Minerals," *American Journal of Clinical Nutrition,* Vol. 9, p. 550, 1961.

says, "From such natural sources one gets a better *balanced* ration of *all* these B-complex vitamins than by taking individual synthetic vitamins or 'enriched' foods to which large quantities of some and none of the others may have been added. There is considerable evidence to prove that the relative proportions of nature's mixtures of B vitamins in foods are those best adapted for promoting health." [2]

The best way to shoot for an optimal intake of the B-complex vitamins is to use daily one or more of the B-complex foods recommended by Dr. Bogert. Let's take a close look at these foods that are so teeming with B-complex vitamins.

ORGAN MEATS

One would expect that the liver which is the "chemical workshop of the body" would contain large quantities of the B-complex vitamins in addition to other vitamins and minerals. A glance at our Food Table will show that three ounces of beef liver contain 14 per cent of the allowance for B_1, and 188 per cent of the B_2 allowance. In addition they contain 28 per cent of the protein allowance, 36 per cent of the vitamin C allowance, 66 per cent of the iron allowance, and 910 per cent of the vitamin A allowance! Liver ranks higher than any other food in its concentration of so many essential nutrients. A wise homemaker will find many ways to prepare it. Besides the usual frying, it can be ground up into a tasty liver loaf, or included in stews.

Organ meats are often neglected and hence are real bargains at the meat counter. If price were based on vitamin and mineral values, and steak is worth a dollar a pound, you should have to pay about fifty-six

2. L. Jean Bogert, *Nutrition and Physical Fitness*, 6th ed., pp. 260-261. (Philadelphia: W. B. Saunders Company, 1954.)

dollars a pound for liver. The Vitamin-Mineral Index of liver is fifty-six times that of steak. Yet lamb and pork liver can often be bought at less than half the cost of steak. Other organ meats that are considerably more nutritious than steaks and muscle meats are kidney, heart, and brains. For example, steak has a Vitamin-Mineral Index of 2; kidneys have an Index of 33; heart, 14; brains, 12. Most cookbooks show various ways to fix these often overlooked but economical meats. Sautéed kidneys, brains and eggs, braised heart, and various casseroles may be deliciously prepared from these unusually nutritious organ meats.

WHEAT GERM

Wheat germ offers you a remarkable package of B vitamins, protein, minerals, and unsaturated fatty acids. I like everything about it except the name—too bad it isn't known as "Heart of Wheat" or something more esthetic. A wheat grain has three parts. The outer bran layer is often made into breakfast food; the inner part is refined into white flour; and the heart from which the new plant germinates is called the "germ" of the wheat. Wheat-germ oil is also loaded with linoleic acid and vitamin E—it is by far the richest source of vitamin E. As you will recall, the protein in wheat germ is a complete one that ranks with steak.

Wheat germ makes a handy breakfast cereal with bananas or other fruit added. It is a delicious hot cereal when lightly simmered in milk. Many people like the extra flavor and nutrition it adds to bread, biscuits, muffins, meatloaf, stews, and soups. Keep it refrigerated, for like most unusually nutritious foods, it will spoil easily.

YEAST

Whenever I think of yeast, I remember someone who feels that he owes his high level of health today to this superlative source of all the B vitamins. A few years ago, Carl's heart began to skip beats. He went to a doctor and the irregular beats appeared on an electrocardiogram. He was told that there was nothing organically wrong with him and that he had "a nervous heart." These attacks had gradually been getting worse over a period of ten years since Carl had been discharged from the Army. He was given Nembutal capsules to help him get through the times his heart would act up.

Carl told me that he dreaded going to bed at night. With the deep circles under his eyes, he looked as though he hadn't slept for weeks. He said he would get up in the morning more tired than when he went to bed. He was terrified when his heart seemed to stop momentarily and then begin again. He would lie there at night on his bed, hour after hour, with sweat running off his body. Sometimes his arms were numb and difficult to move. He was tired most of the time and would easily become irritated.

I told him that while we couldn't be sure exactly what his problem was, I knew that a program directed toward optimal nutrition was usually helpful in enabling the body to increase its resistance to most troubles. He usually ate a good diet of fresh meats, dairy products, vegetables, and fruits, and by usual standards he was not low in B vitamins. However, since the lack of B vitamins is sometimes associated with heart irregularities, I suggested that he add brewer's yeast to his usual diet. Yeast contains all of the B vitamins and is the richest source of most of them.

For three weeks his intake of B_1 and B_2 through

yeast totaled about 250 per cent of the recommended daily allowance. He noticed that he could sleep a little better, but since he did not like yeast, he decided to stop using it. During the next two weeks he did not sleep as well. I was able to get him to begin again with the yeast. I explained to him that sometimes it takes the body a little while to restock and rebuild. Just as health is not usually lost overnight, so it cannot be regained overnight. Two weeks later he reported to me that he was sleeping much better and that his heart was skipping less. Greatly encouraged, he boosted his B_1 and B_2 intake through yeast to about 700 per cent of the allowance. One month later he reported that he was sleeping "like a log" and the dreaded skipping of heartbeats had disappeared. At the end of three months, the dark circles under his eyes were gone and he had a smile and a cheery disposition that were a joy to see.

A year later he asked me whether it would be all right for him to stop using yeast. I told him that he could stop the yeast provided he continued to eat each day at least one food high in the B complex, such as liver or wheat germ. About one month later he reported something that surprised me. His heart was beating irregularly again, but not as bad as before. He began using yeast again, and within ten days the heart symptoms disappeared. Apparently his need for B vitamins is unusually high. He has now decided that optimal nutrition for him must include two to four heaping tablespoons of yeast per day.

YEAST IS THE RICHEST SOURCE OF B VITAMINS

Ounce for ounce, yeast is by far the richest source of B vitamins known. A special yeast has been developed which is designed to meet human nutritional requirements. This is a *torula* food yeast with an unusually fine balance of B vitamins. If you compare this yeast with ordinary yeast (see the Food Table), you will find that it is far richer in vitamins B_1 and B_2. It is 50 per cent protein and it also has small amounts of unsaturated fat. It stores well without refrigeration.

Unfortunately, many people have been prejudiced against yeast. Back in the 1930's, live cake yeast was tried by many people, but the taste was terrible. Nutritionists no longer recommend this type of yeast in live form. Live yeasts will grow in your intestines and steal B vitamins from you. The only yeast recommended by nutritionists today is called "dried brewer's yeast." This yeast has been subjected to sufficient heat to kill the yeast cells and to crack the cell walls so that B vitamins are readily available for digestion. Baker's yeast, which is *live yeast*, should never be eaten unless cooked. Baking or cooking kills the live yeast cells. "Debittered" dried brewer's yeast has been used for making beer and has been salvaged afterward. Its B-vitamin content will be less than the primary dried brewer's yeast that has not been used for beer making. Yeast tablets are usually less potent and more expensive than the powdered yeast.

I have found that Europeans are more accustomed to taking yeast than Americans. Many enjoy its taste. Most Americans think of yeast (if they think of it at all) as a rather bad-tasting substance—and many yeasts are. The better powdered food yeasts are quite palatable when mixed with certain foods. Try them with a glass of tomato juice or V-8 juice. Lime or lemon adds to the flavor. Powdered yeast blends nicely with peanut butter. Carrot juice almost completely masks the taste. Many housewives find that they can add yeast to soups, stews, casseroles, and breads without affecting the taste of these foods.

GO EASY AT FIRST

If you are not used to taking yeast, it is important that you begin cautiously. Start with one-half of a level teaspoon in a glass of vegetable, tomato, or other juice. You will probably not be able to taste it at all. When you are not accustomed to using yeast, its powerhouse of B vitamins may stimulate bacilli in your intestines to produce large amounts of gas that can be uncomfortable. At the beginning, it has a laxative effect if you take too much. If you start with one-half of a level teaspoon the first day and gradually double it every other day for a week, you will probably be able to avoid these effects completely. If gas is produced, cut back your quantity of yeast by one-half and gradually increase it again the next day.

If you use alcoholic drinks, B vitamin-rich foods are especially important to you. These vitamins are essential to burning alcohol in your body. One of the best hangover cures I have heard of is a triple hooker of yeast downed immediately on getting up. This was reported to me by a man who downed a fifth of rum per night on a two-week's vacation in Nassau. The morning after (when there was too little blood in his alcohol stream) he was headachey indeed until he got about one-half cup of yeast in him. (He was accustomed to using yeast.) He reported that within an hour, all hangover was gone and he was ready for another night of celebration. He has tested this sufficiently often to know that it works dependably—for him. Such quantities of alcohol (even when chased by yeast) are definitely not a part of optimal nutrition. A fifth of rum contains 1,843 empty calories.

Yeast may stimulate intestinal health. The B vitamins in the yeast spark the movement of lazy intestines. Drugstore laxatives work by irritating the intestines, by flushing large amounts of water into them, or in other ways that can be upsetting to the body. The proper use of yeast can stimulate natural bowel action and in many cases eliminate the need for harsh laxatives. Bad breath and a heavy white coat on the tongue usually disappear soon, too.

RICE BRAN OR RICE POLISH

A fourth food unusually rich in the B-complex vitamins is rice bran or rice polish. This is the hull that is removed when white rice is milled. When we refine some foods, we separate the more nutritious portions from the less nutritious part. Often the part containing most of the vitamins and minerals is given to animals and the less nutritious used for human consumption. This happens, for example, when sugar cane is refined— man usually ends up eating white sugar that is pure calories and little else. The nutritious concentration of vitamins and minerals that is set aside is called "black-strap molasses." Most of this goes to animals who must be kept healthy to be profitable. When wheat is refined, the more nutritious wheat germ often goes to animals and the less nutritious white flour is eaten by humans.

Similarly, when rice is processed, the outer layer, or bran, is set aside, and the inner portion containing few B vitamins is polished to a shiny white and sold for table use. Only one ounce of this bran furnishes 48 per cent of the daily allowance of vitamin B_1. When white rice is given a final buffing, the resulting polish is blown away and accumulated in a bin. One ounce of this polish is loaded with 41 per cent of the daily allowance for B_1.

Although rice bran and rice polish are available in one-pound packages, I usually rely upon organ meats, wheat germ, and yeast for my B-complex vitamins. An ingenious housewife could, however, use rice bran or polish to enrich breads, stews, soups, casseroles, and other dishes.

It should be emphasized that while most foods contain small amounts of B vitamins, only liver, wheat germ, yeast, and rice bran and polish are extremely rich sources of these energy-releasing vitamins. In my own program of optimal nutrition, I use at least two of these each day and on many days I manage to include three of them.

B VITAMINS AND STRESS

"The true requirements for a given vitamin," Dr. Stanley Davidson points out, "are likely to vary very much from one individual to another." In addition to individual variation, both physical and mental stress may skyrocket your need for certain vitamins of the B complex. The heavy burden of pregnancy and nursing increases the requirements of mothers for these vitamins as well as for most other nutrients. You will note in the "Recommended Allowances for Various Groups" on page 216 that pregnant and nursing women require higher B_1 and B_2 totals. Other stresses that can increase your need for certain B vitamins are fever, infection, surgery, overwork, and psychological tension.

Many people have found that their ability to handle business and personal problems is increased when they double or triple their intake of foods richest in the B-complex vitamins. While writing this book, I was unable to lay aside my other activities. I found it necessary to get up at six o'clock in the morning and write for two to three hours. After a day's work, I began again at six in the evening and often worked until midnight.

Day after day I maintained a 15- to 18-hour work schedule. On the few days when I was too busy to include generous amounts of liver, wheat germ, and yeast in my diet, I found it difficult to continue working efficiently until midnight. On days when I included all three of these in my diet, I was often able to work beyond midnight with a high energy level. Only the thought that I planned to get up at six in the morning made me stop.

B VITAMINS MAY BE LOST IN COOKING

Most cooks are geniuses at destroying B vitamins. It must be remembered that B-complex vitamins are *water soluble* and therefore rapidly dissolve when soaked in water. Boiling is the most vicious type of soaking and removes even more B vitamins. The next chapter will describe a method of cooking vegetables that improves their flavor and permits practically no loss of these vitamins.

In addition to the losses due to soaking and boiling, some B vitamins can be destroyed in other ways. For example, vitamin B_1 is destroyed by heat, especially in an alkaline solution. Baking soda added to water in which vegetables are boiled will destroy it even faster than boiling in plain water. Vitamin B_2 is resistant to heat but may be destroyed by light. Milk that was left on a doorstep in direct sunlight in clear bottles for two hours was found to lose from 54 per cent to 68 per cent of this vitamin. Many dairies prevent this loss by selling milk in colored bottles.

The figures in our Food Table are for foods that have not been mishandled. The National Research Council clearly states that their recommended allowances "do not allow for losses due to storage, cooking, or serving. Provision must be made for these losses in diet planning." [3] *This is another reason for taking the high road to optimal nutrition.*

B VITAMINS ARE NONTOXIC

Since B vitamins are water soluble, they are excreted in the urine whenever they are oversupplied. This means that they are nontoxic unless taken in fantastic amounts in pill form. Rats given 25,000 times the daily requirement of vitamin B_1 showed no ill effects; nor did mice given 1,000 times the minimum requirement of B_2. You apparently have everything to gain by treating your body to a generous intake of these energy-releasing vitamins when you get them from foods.

It should always be borne in mind that water-soluble vitamins (including vitamin C and most of the B complex) are not stored in the body in any substantial amounts. All you can do is to saturate your tissues with these nutrients. Saturation means that your daily intake has been at such a high level that each cell and tissue has absorbed the maximum that it can. A sheet of cardboard, for example, will not store water like a bottle, but it can be saturated with water so that the fibers of the paper will hold the maximum possible.

OPTIMAL NUTRITION AND "ENRICHMENT"

When the germ of wheat and corn is removed, the resulting white flour and corn meal are deprived of many nutrients, including much complete protein, un-

3. *Recommended Dietary Allowances, Revised 1958,* Publication 589, p. 27. (Washington, D.C.: National Academy of Sciences— National Research Council, 1958.)

saturated fat, most of the vitamins of the B complex, and most of the minerals. To use the label "enriched," the manufacturer must restore the B_1, B_2, niacin, and iron. These grains are "enriched" only in the sense that you are enriched by losing a dollar and finding a quarter. There is no doubt that the synthetic vitamins added to white flour, corn meal, and some cereals help folks who live on poor diets of refined foods. But if you are striving for optimal nutrition, you will have no use for this type of "enrichment," for most of your foods will be untouched by what Dr. Samuel Soskin bitterly called "the evils of modern food refinement." [4] We can approve of genuine enrichment when it is judiciously done without stealing nutrients first. This is the case when vitamin D is added to milk, vitamin A is added to margarine, vitamin E is added to a food to retard rancidity, or iodine is added to table salt.

WHAT ABOUT PILLS?

During the past two decades, the use of self-administered vitamin and mineral pills and capsules has soared. I am often asked, "Why should I bother learning about foods when I can simply take a ten-cent vitamin and mineral pill each day?" I wish the attainment of optimal health were that simple. How wonderful it would be if we could simply swallow a pill or capsule and then choose foods on a basis of taste and habit.

Numerous short-term experiments have shown that for most people these vitamin-mineral preparations add nothing to physical fitness. No one knows whether the long-term effects are good, bad, or indifferent. It's my conviction the highest level of health for humans does

4. Samuel Soskin and Rachmiel Levine, "Carbohydrate Malnutrition," from Norman Jolliffe, F. F. Tisdall, Paul A. Cannon, eds., *Clinical Nutrition*, pp. 224-226. (New York: Hoeber Medical Division, Harper & Row, Publishers, Inc., 1950.)

not come out of a bottle—unless it is a bottle of milk. There are far more nutritional values in natural foods than in any vitamin-mineral preparations now available. A dime's worth of pills may buy a dime's worth of health. I personally will settle for nothing less than an approach to optimal nutrition through the finest choice of the finest foods.

NUTRIENTS YET TO BE DISCOVERED

When animals are tested with toxic drugs or injected with infectious bacilli, they sometimes show a need for nutrients that are yet unknown. For example, the resistance of mice to an infection was considerably increased by an unknown nutrient in wheat germ. Scientists tried all known nutrients to duplicate the resistance that was given to these animals by wheat germ, but they were unsuccessful.

In other experiments in which animals were given large quantities of toxic drugs, it was found that liver was a potent source of unknown nutrients that gave a degree of protection against these drugs. Liver was also found to contain unknown nutrients that prolonged the survival of rats that were subjected to X-rays. In addition to liver and wheat germ, it was found that kidney, soybeans, and yeast contain unidentified nutrients.[5] These unknown nutrients, of course, are not available in synthetic vitamin pills and are probably present only in insignificant quantities in most foods that have been refined.

If you aren't willing to intelligently select natural foods of high quality, you cannot expect to approach an optimal level of health, energy, and longevity. When you follow the program of nutrition recommended in this book, you will have no need for vitamin or min-

5. *Nutrition Reviews*, Vol. 13, p. 35, 1955.

eral supplements unless fighting illness. Vitamin D, described in Chapter 14, is a possible exception. Nature expected us to get this vitamin from sunshine, but some folks stay out of the sun as much as possible.

IT TAKES TEAMWORK

I think of organ meats, wheat germ, and yeast as energy-releasing foods that can help you toward a higher level of health. However, it is misleading to expect these foods by themselves to bring energy or increased health —just as hundred-octane gas will not by itself increase the power of a car engine. The engine must be in sound operating condition. Good lubricating oil must minimize friction; water in the radiator must cool the engine; the battery and generator must supply optimal electrical power; the spark plugs must be clean, etc. Hundred-octane gas is only a part of the team. It is, however, a vital part, for the engine won't run well on kerosene any more than our bodies will operate well if we eat junk.

Each individual nutrient is only a spoke in the wheel of health. It cannot by itself produce any of the benefits discussed in this book. But in cooperation with a nearly optimal supply of the other nutrients, and provided your bodily machine is structurally and functionally in good condition, these nutrients can do their job in bringing you greater energy, less disease, and more zest-filled years.

The health of your body is to some extent interwoven with your mental goings-on. The performance of a car is not affected by whether it is delivering a thumbtack or carrying the President of the United States. Unlike a car, your physical equipment will do its best only when highly motivated by interesting ego-satisfying activities. Your reaction to your total life situation —your motivating goals, your emotional relationships, your happiness—these and countless other parts of your thought-life continuously interact with the performance of your body. It can make a lot of difference in our energy level whether we are fishing or just cutting bait.

Chapter 13

VERSATILE VITAMIN C

On November 4, 1740, Lord Anson sailed from England to the New World with six ships manned by 961 stalwart seamen. During those days the food on board consisted largely of salt-cured meat and biscuits with no fresh fruit or vegetables containing vitamin C. Sailors were concerned about sea monsters lurking over the distant horizons, but the lack of vitamin C in their diet proved to be far more dangerous than all the terrors of the sea. Six months later, when Lord Anson's fleet reached America, two-thirds of the crew had died of scurvy and three ships had been abandoned. After he had been gone a year, scurvy had so reduced his crew that he had to abandon two more ships. When he returned to England about three and a half years later, five of his six ships and more than 80 per cent of his crew had been lost through scurvy.[1] In 1757 Lind proved that lemons would prevent scurvy and "lime juice" became a part of the diet of British sailors—that is the origin of the nickname "limeys."

1. R. Walter, *Lord Anson's Voyage Round the World, 1740-44.* Abridged and annotated by Pack, S. W. C. (London: Penguin Books, 1947.)

We know today that vitamin C is richly supplied by all citrus fruit. This vitamin is also called "ascorbic acid" in recognition of its effectiveness in curing scurvy.

VITAMIN C MAKES INTERCELLULAR CEMENT

Have you ever wondered what keeps teeth tightly cemented in your jaw bone? What makes the miles and miles of your veins, arteries, and capillaries watertight so that blood does not leak out? What keeps muscles firmly attached to your bones? The answer is that your body is held together by a cement-like substance called "collagen" which cannot be made if vitamin C is unavailable. Collagen is often referred to as "intercellular cement." But there is a striking difference between the permanence of the cement that holds your body together and the cement that is used in laying the bricks of a building. Once a brick is laid, that cement can never be used again. But when you are short on vitamin C, your body will remove the collagen that holds you together. Dr. Mary L. Dodd of Pennsylvania State University has pointed out that if vitamin C is deficient, "the cementing material is missing, and the cells literally seem to fall apart." [2] Fortunately scurvy is rare today, but signs of a deficiency in vitamin C are far from rare. Most animals make their own vitamin C, but guinea pigs, monkeys, and men *are dependent on their diet* for this versatile vitamin.

A mirror will quickly tell you if your gums are in good condition. They should be pink, not red; firm, not swollen; they should join tightly to your teeth. If they are spongy, puffy, or red where they join your teeth, you may have a deficiency of vitamin C. If this

2. *Food, The Yearbook of Agriculture 1959*, p. 152, Department of Agriculture. (Washington, D.C.: U.S. Government Printing Office.)

condition continues, gums may look like bags of blood and teeth may become loose and eventually come out. More teeth are lost by adults through deterioration of the gums than through decay. When your body is liberally supplied with vitamin C, your teeth will tend to remain tightly cemented to your jawbone. Gingivitis, unless due to improper brushing or other factors, will usually be cured within several months when the diet provides generous amounts of vitamin C.

Another sign that vitamin C may be low in your diet is a tendency toward bruises. If you are deficient in this vitamin, your blood vessels may lose some of their flexibility so that a bump or blow can easily break them. This rupture of tiny blood vessels permits some blood to escape into the tissues where it shows as a bruise. Women who are low on vitamin C are particularly susceptible to bruising. Frequently bumps that are not even hard enough to be remembered will make bruises on their legs. As Dr. Bogert expressed it, ". . . blood vessel walls become more fragile and are likely to 'spring a leak.' . . ." In extreme vitamin C deficiency, even the slight pressure from clothes can cause bruises. If you take a pencil and write on the skin, the resulting breakage of vitamin-C-starved blood vessels will show up as though you had written in red ink.

FOR HEALING AND GROWTH

When vitamin C is not available in the body, wounds will not heal. In scurvy, old wounds may break open as the body steals collagen that was previously laid down. Although scurvy is rare among adult Americans, it is interesting to consider an account of Lord Anson's voyage that tells of the results when the body withdraws this cementing substance during a *severe* deficiency of vitamin C: ". . . one of the invalids on board the *Centurion*, who had been wounded about fifty years before at the battle of the Boyne, for though he was cured soon after, and had continued well for a great number of years past, yet on his being attacked by the scurvy, his wounds, in the progress of his disease, broke out afresh and appeared as if they had never been healed: nay, what is still more astonishing, the callus of a broken bone, which had been completely formed for a long time, was found to be hereby dissolved, and the fracture seemed as if it had never been consolidated." [3]

Vitamin C has a large part to play in the growth of bones. When it is undersupplied, there is damage to the cartilage in the growing ends of bones. They may slip apart at the joints due to the lack of supporting cartilage. Calcium is a mineral that gives strength to bones. Along with vitamin D, vitamin C is necessary for calcium to be deposited and held in bones and teeth.

Although adult scurvy is rare in the United States, infantile scurvy is sometimes seen. Human milk is well supplied with vitamin C—it contains three to four times more than cow's milk. Scurvy may develop a few months after breast feeding is stopped if vitamin C is not available. Unfortunately, first symptoms are hidden. As the infant's bones stop growing properly, joints begin to swell and walking and sitting become painful. The child lies on its back in order to avoid pain when he moves his legs. The front ends of his ribs are sore and breathing may be difficult. Since being lifted is painful, the infant may cry when he is handled or even approached. Fortunately, all this may be changed in three to four days when vitamin C is supplied.

Children who are low in vitamin C are irritable, slightly retarded in growth, and lacking in stamina.

3. R. Walter, *op. cit.*

These conditions are promptly corrected when they are given orange juice or other food that provides this important nutrient. A lack of vitamin C in older children and adults is often associated with listlessness, loss of energy, lack of endurance, fleeting pains in the legs and joints which are often mistaken for rheumatism, muscular weakness, and a poor level of overall health.

Dr. S. B. Wolbach found the following physiological changes due to a shortage of vitamin C:

1. Hemorrhages may occur anywhere in the body.
2. Profound changes may take place in the teeth and gums.
3. The growing ends of bones may become deformed.
4. Bones fall apart due to loss of supporting cartilage.
5. The heart can become enlarged and the heart muscles may be damaged.
6. The muscles throughout the body may degenerate causing extreme weakness and even death.
7. The blood may become anemic because of the destruction of blood-forming cells in the bone marrow and the loss of blood by hemorrhage.
8. The bones may sometimes become so soft that they break spontaneously because of the lack of calcium.
9. The sex organs and other glandular tissues may degenerate.[4]

Dr. Sherman has indicated that vitamin C may assist in deferring the process of aging. An optimal supply of this vitamin can help you feel young, look young, and act young.

4. S. B. Wolbach, "The Pathological Changes Resulting from Vitamin Deficiency," *Journal of the American Medical Association*, Vol. 108, pp. 7-13, 1937.

FOR FIGHTING INFECTION

Although other vitamins help you in a general way to build health and thus avoid infection, vitamin C has a specific role in fighting infection. This brave vitamin stands ever ready to sacrifice itself to fight invading bacteria. Doctors Menton and King fed guinea pigs various amounts of vitamin C and then infected them with diphtheria toxin. The animals that had the least vitamin C suffered the most from the ravages of diphtheria even though they showed no signs of scurvy. Animals that had a very liberal intake showed far greater resistance.

Experiments were conducted with vitamin C in an English school. Over a six-month period the boys on a low intake of vitamin C averaged twice as many days in the infirmary, compared with those who received an adequate intake.[5]

It is known that your body can use up enormous quantities of vitamin C when under stress. Even a slight cold can deplete your blood of this vitamin. It is also used in large amounts when your body is troubled by allergy, infection, or invaded by drugs or toxic chemicals. Even an aspirin knocks out some vitamin C. Any damage to your body such as a burn, fracture, or surgical operation will probably deplete your blood of vitamin C unless you immediately and continually provide yourself with very large quantities of this fleeting vitamin.

Unfortunately, vitamin C is not stored in the body. All you can do is saturate your tissues. Saturation is the point at which all of your tissues have soaked up as much as they can retain, and any vitamin C taken above this level will be promptly excreted in the urine.

5. *Nutrition Reviews*, Vol. 1, p. 202, 1943.

The need for vitamin C is apparently so great during some illnesses that incredibly large quantities may be taken without saturating the tissues. It is not toxic even when taken hourly in large quantities by synthetic pills.

In 1936, Dr. Szent-Gyorgy, the discoverer of vitamin C, found substances in oranges which interact with vitamin C in decreasing capillary bleeding and prolonging the life of guinea pigs. For a while they were known as vitamin P, but this name was dropped in 1950. These substances, rutin and hesperidin complex, are now called "bioflavonoids." It has been found that they have a protective effect when dogs and rats are subjected to injury by X-rays.[6] Their role in human nutrition is not known at this time. If they eventually prove to be a part of optimal human nutrition, you will be well supplied with bioflavonoids if you get a generous amount of vitamin C from fresh fruits and vegetables.

VITAMIN C IS NEEDED DAILY

Keeping your body saturated with water-soluble B and C vitamins is a day-to-day affair. Experiments with guinea pigs have shown that when these animals were given a supply of vitamin C once a week, it was only about one-fourth as effective as when they received the same amount of vitamin C divided into daily doses. Similar tests with vitamin A showed that weekly intakes were just as effective as daily ones because vitamin A is easily stored in the liver. Dr. E. N. Todhunter ran an experiment in which she gave people two-thirds of the recommended daily allowance of vitamin C at one

6. J. B. Field and P. E. Rekers, "Studies of the Effects of Flavonoids on Roentgen Irradiation Disease. II. Comparison of the Protective Influence of Some Flavonoids and Vitamin C in Dogs," *Journal of Clinical Investigation*, Vol. 28, p. 746, 1949.

time.[7] The amount in the blood began to increase in about thirty minutes. It reached a maximum in ninety minutes. It was excreted rapidly by the kidneys, and three to four hours later the vitamin C in the blood was the same as before the experiment. If you stopped your intake of this vitamin, your present blood level of vitamin C would drop 50 per cent in sixteen days. At the end of ten weeks you would have none in your blood plasma.[8]

If you want your blood to be as rich as possible in this vitamin, it is important that you eat vitamin C foods several times per day. An orange eaten morning, noon, and night would for most people in good health maintain a saturation or near saturation level of vitamin C. Since citric acid in oranges, lemons, and limes may, over many years, etch the enamel of your teeth, it may be desirable to wash your mouth out with water after eating citrus fruits if they are used several times a day.

An excessive amount of water can flush B and C vitamins out of your body. Experiments have shown that an overuse of water can give you a deficiency in these vitamins even though your diet meets adequate standards. However, *water is probably the most important of all nutrients*. The lack of it can result in death much quicker than with any other nutrient. Adequate water keeps the kidneys flushed out and will help prevent fatigue during hard physical work. The ancient Greek formula of moderation—avoid too little or too much—should be the watchword here. For healthy people, thirst is usually a good guide.

7. E. N. Todhunter, R. C. Robbins, and J. A. McIntosh, "The Rate of Increase of Blood Plasma Ascorbic Acid After Ingestion of Ascorbic Acid (Vitamin C)," *Journal of Nutrition*, Vol. 23, pp. 309-319, 1942.

8. C. J. Farmer, "Some Aspects of Vitamin C Metabolism," *Federation Proceedings*, Vol. 3, p. 179, 1944.

FRAGILE VITAMIN C

Of all the vitamins, vitamin C is used in the largest quantity by the body, yet it is the most fragile. Losses between the farm and your kitchen may be great. For example, carrots and broccoli can lose 44 per cent of their vitamin C just sitting for two days at room temperature. When broccoli is kept in a refrigerator for two days, there is only an 8 per cent loss. When placed on crushed ice there is practically no loss. Tomatoes hold this vitamin better at room temperature and may only lose 12 per cent in two days.

If you wish to have ample supplies of this vitamin, it is important to buy only the freshest and finest produce. Poor quality or wilted vegetables contain less vitamin C than the amounts shown in our Food Table. Dr. Van Duyne found that three and one-half ounces of freshly picked broccoli could supply as little as 121 per cent or as much as 229 per cent of the recommended allowance. Fully ripe vegetables that receive the most sunlight will tend to be richest in vitamin C.

A small back yard garden may be an excellent way to provide your family with crisp, fresh greens. The salads I have enjoyed most were made from leaves that were growing only fifteen minutes before. If your garden space is limited, by all means concentrate on salad greens, for these are most likely to suffer by the inevitable delays of marketing. A plot about ten feet square (sowed as a bed instead of in rows) can raise enough for an average-size family.

I don't have much of a green thumb. When I planted my garden, the turnips were the only vegetables that survived the uncertainties of sprouting and the onslaught of insects. I was delighted to find that young, fresh turnip greens make a delicious salad. I cut the tender young turnip leaves when they were six to eight inches high. They are like crisp lettuce and lack the strong flavor associated with cooked turnip greens. You may be surprised if you compare lettuce and turnip greens in the Food Table. Lettuce has a Vitamin-Mineral Index of 39; turnip greens hit the gong with an Index of 207!

To preserve vitamin C in the fruits and vegetables you buy, put them in the refrigerator as soon as possible. Some vitamin C is destroyed when foods are crushed, ground, or bruised. When chopping vegetables for salads, use a sharp knife. Some vitamin C is destroyed when it comes into contact with iron, brass, or copper. It has been found that coleslaw mixed with a steel kitchen fork lost about 13 per cent more vitamin C than when mixed with a silver fork. Straining orange juice through a brass or copper sieve filters out some vitamin C as well as the seeds.

Like the B vitamins, vitamin C is soluble in water and will leap out when vegetables are soaked. It is also destroyed by heat—especially in an alkaline solution such as soda. Even contact with air or light will hasten its destruction. To retain maximum vitamin C, an orange should be peeled and sliced into as large pieces as you can chew. If you prefer juice, however, it is best to use it as quickly as possible, although not too much vitamin C will be lost overnight if you keep it cold and covered with as little air space as possible between the juice and the cover. Unlike other fruits and vegetables, citrus fruits hold this vitamin well when stored. Even canning and processing *if carefully done* will retain 90 per cent of the original vitamin C.

Charles Dana Gibson's cook once asked him, "The potatoes, sir, do you want them in the jackets or in the nude?" When potatoes are boiled as long as forty minutes in their jackets, there is only a 10 per cent loss of

vitamin C. When boiled "in the nude," 30 per cent is
lost. When they are held overnight after cooking, they
may lose 65 per cent of this vitamin. Vegetables held
on a restaurant steam table for hours may lose almost
all their vitamin C.[9]

STEAMING RETAINS NUTRITION AND FLAVOR

For dinner one evening I had three vegetables—all
of which were cooked without even dirtying one pot.
The turnip greens and broccoli were a mouthwatering
bright green; the carrots were bright orange. They had a
delicious flavor that is never found in boiled vegetables.
Surprisingly enough, they were all cooked together in
the same pot, touching each other, but there was no
mingling of flavors. Sounds almost unbelievable, doesn't
it? These were cooked by steaming in an ordinary pot
—no pressure cooker was used. When carrots are
boiled fifteen minutes, they lose 40 per cent of their
vitamin C. Eleven per cent is destroyed and 29 per cent
dissolves into the cooking water. When carrots are
steamed for fifteen minutes, only 14 per cent of this
vitamin is lost.[10]

If you want your vegetables to retain almost all
their vitamins and minerals; if you want them to have
a mouthwatering look and to taste unusually delicious;
if you don't enjoy washing pots and pans—steaming
is for you. Pressure cookers will do the job, but they
are too much trouble for most people. Any ordinary
saucepan with a tight-fitting lid can be used to steam
your vegetables. It is necessary to have a metal shelf that

9. From *Vitamin and Mineral Content of Certain Foods as
Affected by Home Preparation.* Miscellaneous Publication No. 628.
(Washington, D.C.: U.S. Department of Agriculture, 1948.)
10. F. Fenton, D. K. Tressler, S. C. Camp, and C. G. King,
"Losses of Vitamin C During Boiling and Steaming of Carrots,"
Food Research, Vol. 3, pp. 403-408, 1938.

fits in the pan with small holes in it to let the steam through. This shelf is placed about two inches above the bottom of the pot, and it holds the food *above* the boiling water. The pot is filled with about an inch of water and this is brought to a boil before vegetables are put in.

When vegetables are put into live steam, the enzymes in the plants are rapidly destroyed before they have a chance to do much damage to the vitamin C. While cooking, the water boils merrily away in the bottom of the pan but it does not get to the vegetables. You will find that the softer vegetables such as tomatoes need only four or five minutes while others will require ten to fifteen minutes. You can start the carrots first, then add broccoli after five minutes and then tomatoes after another five minutes. A few more minutes and they are all ready to serve. I like most vegetables to retain a little crunchiness after cooking, so I am careful not to overcook.

Steaming trivets with adjustable sides that will fit into various-sized saucepans can be bought in many department stores. These are usually made from aluminum or stainless steel and are perforated like a colander to let the steam come up from the bottom of the pan. You can cook four or five vegetables at the same time with one of these steamers. Onions may be in contact with more delicately flavored vegetables and there will never be a mingling of flavors because all of the vitamins, minerals, and other nutrients stay where they belong and are not dissolved out by boiling water. Unthawed frozen vegetables may simply be placed in the steamer and the live steam will cook them in the most nutritious and delicious way.

For busy modern folks who are in a hurry, this method of cooking vegetables is a godsend. It will spoil you, though. I have found that after delicious steamed vegetables, I am unable to enjoy vegetables that have been boiled. They not only look flat, but also taste flat. When bananas are steamed (not in the nude), heat changes the starch to sugar and they have a most delicious flavor. If you have never tried steaming vegetables, you have a real treat in store for you.

THE ROAD TO OPTIMAL VITAMIN C

The National Research Council recommends that children up to three years have a vitamin C total of 47 per cent as computed from our Food Table. To meet heavy needs during growth, this is gradually increased so that a ten- to twelve-year-old will get the same amount as an adult man—a vitamin C total of 100 per cent. You will note in the "Recommended Allowances for Various Groups" shown on page 216 that teenage boys from sixteen to nineteen years need a vitamin C total of 133 per cent.

It is especially important that mothers have a good intake of this vitamin. During the second half of pregnancy, they recommend a vitamin C intake of 133 per cent. While nursing, the vitamin C total should be maintained at 200 per cent. The National Research Council states regarding their recommendations for vitamin C, "They are not 'saturation' values, since more generous intakes result in distinctly higher concentrations in the tissues." [11]

Since you use this vitamin rapidly, saturating your body with vitamin C is like filling a glass that has a small opening in the bottom. You've got to keep filling it to keep the level high. But once it is full, any excess overflows and is lost. When your tissues are not saturated,

11. *Recommended Dietary Allowances, Revised 1958,* Publication 589, p. 16. (Washington, D.C.: National Academy of Sciences—National Research Council, 1958.)

some of the vitamin C will be retained in your body. When saturation is achieved, almost all of the extra vitamin C you eat will be rapidly excreted. Dr. E. N. Todhunter found that saturation can be obtained if your vitamin C total as shown in your Nutrition Analysis Form is equal to your weight in pounds.[12] She suggested that your vitamin C foods be distributed throughout the day. In other words, if you weigh 180 pounds, your vitamin C total should be 180 per cent to maintain saturation. Other researchers have found that mothers during pregnancy and while nursing need a vitamin C score of 400 per cent to achieve a saturation level.

Thus scientific evidence available today indicates that you can probably maintain saturation with a daily vitamin C total (based on our Food Table) that is equal to your weight. However, your day-to-day needs may vary. Vitamin C is easily destroyed both outside and inside your body. It is therefore possible that future research may show long-term optimal benefits from maintaining a daily vitamin C total that is perhaps *double* your weight. A 150-pound man would thus perhaps shoot for a vitamin C total of 300 per cent.

SATURATION UNDER CONDITIONS OF STRESS

Since vitamin C is used in such large quantities under conditions of stress, the amounts mentioned above will only keep your blood saturated with this vitamin under normal conditions. To maintain saturation during illness or injury may require an hourly intake of huge amounts of this vitamin. It is, for example, almost impossible for a person with tuberculosis to stay saturated with this fighting vitamin. When a person with active tuberculosis has a daily vitamin C intake of 1333 per

12. E. N. Todhunter and R. C. Robbins, *Journal of Nutrition,* Vol. 19, p. 263, 1940.

cent, he will only have a blood level that is equivalent to that of most people with a vitamin C total of 100 per cent! [13]

When your body is fighting allergies, chemical poisons, infections, colds, burns, almost all forms of active illness, broken bones, accident damage, surgery, or when you're taking drugs, vitamin C is consumed at a terrific rate. In severe illness, thirty times the recommended daily allowance may be injected into the blood at one time and a blood test a few minutes later may reveal it has been used up immediately. Such large needs cannot usually be met by foods. High potency 500-milligram vitamin C tablets are useful at these times. A vitamin C total of 100 per cent equals 75 milligrams of this vitamin. Thus one 500-milligram tablet furnishes 667 per cent of the recommended allowance.

The Committee on Therapeutic Nutrition of the Food and Nutrition Board of the National Research Council has recommended that during the acute phase of stress the daily intake of vitamin C be increased thirteen to twenty-seven times above the usual allowance (1,000 to 2,000 milligrams). While convalescing, they recommend that the vitamin C total be maintained at 400 per cent (300 milligrams). For burns and other extensive tissue damage and for long-bone fractures, they suggest 1,000 milligrams daily during the acute phase and a vitamin C total of 400 per cent during convalescence (300 milligrams).[14]

I keep a bottle of 500-milligram tablets of vitamin C handy at all times. In some drugstores, vitamin C tablets will run as high as eight dollars per hundred. Cut-rate sources and mail-order firms may offer the

13. Horace R. Getz, "Nutrition and Tuberculosis," *Nutrition Reviews*, Vol. 5, p. 98, 1947.
14. *Therapuetic Nutrition*, publication 234. (Washington, D.C.: National Academy of Sciences—National Research Council, 1952.)

500-milligram tablets for around a dollar-fifty per hundred.

Some mothers wishing to get saturation amounts of vitamin C into their ill children dissolve three 500-milligram tablets in a little hot water and add it to a glass of orange juice. This can be given hourly. Children like it when frozen on sticks so as to make a popsicle. Sometimes fevers are quickly broken by large amounts of vitamin C. Since it is not toxic, and since it is used by the body in huge amounts during illness, it may safely be given in large quantities and any surplus will be rapidly excreted.

Dr. D. Brown found that guinea pigs getting their daily vitamin C through pills showed retarded growth compared with those who obtained this vitamin each day from green cabbage.[15] It would seem that these animals benefited from other nutrients present in the whole natural food. I suggest using synthetic ascorbic acid pills generously when fighting illness, but for your daily nutrition it seems wiser to rely on fruits and vegetables.

15. D. Brown, I. D. Ferguson, and A. G. Ramsey, "Guinea Pigs Reared on a Diet Containing Synthetic Ascorbic Acid," *Journal of Physiology*, Vol. 121, p. 36, 1953.

Chapter 14

VITAMINS D, E, AND K

Many years ago physicians noticed that children who lived in the deep valleys of the Swiss Alps sometimes had severe rickets, whereas children living up in the mountains escaped the bowed legs and protruding ribs of this disease. The doctors rightly guessed that the mountain sunshine had a beneficial effect. We know today that children who lived in the valleys got rickets because the mountains shut out sunshine needed to make vitamin D. The main function of vitamin D is to enable you to build and maintain strong bones. Although nature expects you to make this vitamin in your body, the chances are you are not busy making much of it.

Vitamin D is created when oils in your skin are exposed to the ultraviolet rays of the sun. Unfortunately, this simple method of providing your body with vitamin D does not work well nowadays for some people. We tend to cover our bodies so well that only small areas may be exposed to sunshine. Even then, we usually make a beeline for the shade. Furthermore, the ultraviolet rays of the sun penetrate best through the atmosphere in most of the United States between 10:00 AM and 2:00 PM. They are easily blocked out by clothing, ordinary window glass, smoke, clouds, dust, and pigment in the skin. Reflected light, such as occurs when clouds cover the sun, may produce tiny amounts of vitamin D.

Calcium and phosphorus are the main building blocks that are laid down in a protein framework when bones are formed. All of us know that infants and children are busy building bones, but few are aware that *bone tissues in adults are living structures that are constantly being washed away and rebuilt by the body*. While you read this, there is a very slow disintegration taking place in your bones. If your nutrition is adequate, new bone is constantly being formed. If you get insufficient vitamin D, your bones may become thinner and thinner and will break easily. This is known as adult rickets or osteomalacia.

Suppose you take up a new activity, such as gardening, that places new stresses upon your bones. The new mineralization in your bones that is constantly taking place when your diet is adequate will *gradually* be laid down in such a way as to give them the added strength required for your new activities. Thus your bones are living structures that slowly adapt themselves to your activities and needs.

When you are not well supplied with vitamin D, the amount of calcium and phosphorous in your blood will drop. One reason for this is that vitamin D somehow helps the intestinal wall absorb calcium and phosphorus more readily. It also plays a part in assisting these minerals to be deposited where needed in your bones or teeth. Vitamin D, in common with certain other nutrients, is found to increase both the volume and acidity of your digestive juices which are needed for efficient absorption. Like the other oil-soluble vitamins, vitamin D is best absorbed during a meal when the flow of bile is adequate.

The rapid growth of infants makes this vitamin

especially important. Vitamin D is measured in international units. It has been found that most babies will get by on 150 international units of vitamin D per day. When this is increased to 400 daily, their bones are stronger, and this amount is recommended by the National Research Council. If a growing child is lacking in vitamin D, his permanent teeth may be ruined for the rest of his life. The enamel will be thin, pitted, grooved, and in severe cases, it may even be absent. Mothers sometimes forget the importance of this vitamin. Since it can be stored in the body, some doctors give infants and children a 250,000-unit dose twice a year.

The atomic-bomb tests have filled the atmosphere of the entire world with radioactive strontium 90. It is now present in all of our food, and it is absorbed by our bones. Recent research has shown that a diet high in Vitamin D and calcium gives us the best protection against this tragic part of twentieth-century "civilization." [1]

SOURCES OF VITAMIN D

Sunlight touching the oils in your skin can make vitamin D for you. The whiter your skin, the greater the quantity of skin oil that is irradiated into vitamin D. As we accumulate exposure time, our skin becomes tanned. The darker pigments then begin to screen out some of the ultraviolet rays and thus prevent an oversupply of this vitamin. Perhaps the peoples of Africa developed dark skins to limit their production of vitamin D. Since their skin is such a good filter, little vitamin D is available through sunlight to most Negroes who live in temperate climates.

1. A. E. Sobel, S. Nobel, and P. A. Laurence, *Chemical Engineering News*, Vol. 37, p. 42, 1959.

The best food source of vitamin D is saltwater fish. The oil in the bodies of fish such as herring, salmon, tuna, menhaden, turbot, and sardines contains useful quantities. Three and a half ounces of herring will have a vitamin D content of 1,500 units. One-half cup of salmon supplies 375 to 600 units. Three and a half ounces of canned tuna will have around 250 units.

Vitamin D is highly concentrated in the liver of certain saltwater fish. Cod-liver oil contains a minimum of 400 units per teaspoon plus as much vitamin A as three and a half apricots. Oil from the liver of the bluefin tuna has 600 times more vitamin D than cod-liver oil, plus vitamin A. Only a few drops are needed from products—such as oleum percomorphum—made from the liver of ocean fish that do such a good job of concentrating this vitamin for us.

Once you leave the oily saltwater fish department, vitamin D is quite scarce in the grocery store. Three and a half ounces of liver can contain from 15 to 45 units. Three pats of butter average 12 units and a pint of milk averages 16 units. Eggs are perhaps highest—but it may take fifteen eggs to obtain 400 units per day if the chickens were well supplied with this vitamin.

Because it is so lacking in most foods, the AMA has approved the fortification of milk with vitamin D. To meet their specifications, a quart of milk must contain 400 international units. In some states, vitamin D is available in skim milk. This is a very stable vitamin and there is practically no loss when foods are cooked.

Vitamin D can be made by subjecting plant oils to ultraviolet radiation. Viosterol is produced by this method. It is very concentrated and only a few drops are needed. An ultraviolet lamp may be used in your home as a substitute for sunlight. Sunglasses must be worn to protect your eyes, since these rays can damage the retina of your eyes.

TOXIC LEVELS OF VITAMIN D

Like vitamin A, this vitamin is toxic when used over a long time in extremely large amounts. According to McLester and Darby, "Vitamin D poisoning has been associated with ingestion of 100,000 IU or more of D per day in adults and with 20,000 to 40,000 IU to infants." [2] These dosages must be continued for many months to be toxic.

A 53-year-old woman was treated by her physician with a daily dosage of thyroid, calcium lactate, and 500,000 units of vitamin D. After two years of this enormous dosage, she was "ill and anemic." All symptoms disappeared within three months after this medication was discontinued.[3] The case is mentioned here to give you an idea of the very large margin of safety between the amount we shall recommend and the levels that have been found to be toxic. Vitamin D can do more than prevent disease. In optimal quantities it can help build a higher level of health. Too little or too much should be avoided.

AN APPROACH TO OPTIMAL VITAMIN D

Our distant ancestors probably evolved over a period of millions of years when sunshine was able to bathe their entire bodies and thus provide presumably optimal amounts of vitamin D. Civilization has changed the tune here, as in so many other nutritional matters. Unless you lead an outdoor life, you may be too sheltered from the sun to produce what may be optimal amounts of this vitamin.

2. James S. McLester and William J. Darby, *Nutrition and Diet in Health and Disease*, 6th ed., p. 91. (Philadelphia: W. B. Saunders Company, 1952.)

3. P. Davies, *Annals of Internal Medicine*, Vol. 53, p. 1250, 1960.

Research has shown that normal infants thrive on 400 to 800 units of vitamin D daily. Jeans and Stern found that when normal infants were given 1,500 units or more daily, they had a loss of appetite and did not grow as well as those maintained on a smaller amount. However, with premature infants, more vitamin D is needed—2,000 units daily are recommended by Dr. Edwards A. Park of the Johns Hopkins University School of Medicine.[4]

Numerous studies indicate that the need for vitamin D continues during adolescence. Dr. J. A. Johnston in the *Journal of the American Medical Association* indicated that during the periods of rapid growth at six months and just before puberty, the need for vitamin D is probably twice as great as at any other time of life. During the second half of pregnancy and while nursing, 400 units daily are recommended for women by the National Research Council.

"It is impossible to state the vitamin D requirements exactly," says Dr. L. Jean Bogert. "We can estimate fairly well the amount of it supplied in foods, but there is no way of knowing how much extra vitamin D is made in the body under the influence of sunlight. Since its action is chiefly concerned with the metabolism of bones, which are hidden and relatively inactive tissues, it is difficult to tell whether an adult is or is not getting enough of this vitamin to keep the body in best condition." [5]

Since short-term nutritional research with adults has failed to show as great a need for vitamin D as for growing children, the National Research Council

4. Edwards A. Park, "Vitamin D Malnutrition and Rickets," from Norman Jolliffe, F. F. Tisdall, and Paul R. Cannon, eds., *Clinical Nutrition*, p. 449. (New York: Hoeber Medical Division, Harper & Row, Publishers, Inc., 1950.)

5. L. Jean Bogert, *Nutrition and Physical Fitness*, 6th ed., p. 293. (Philadelphia: W. B. Saunders Company, 1954.)

advises: "The need for supplemental vitamin D by vigorous adults leading a normal life seems to be minimal. For persons working at night and for nuns and others whose habits shield them from the sunlight, as well as for elderly persons, the ingestion of small amounts of vitamin D is desirable. . . . The optimum amount of vitamin D is not known, but [calcium] retention values obtained by some investigators with high dosages of vitamin D seem no greater than those with moderate dosage. On the basis of available evidence, 400 units is probably adequate." [6]

As with other nutrients, exact data on the optimal level of vitamin D for adults is unfortunately not yet available. It is likely, however, that you and I are making far less vitamin D than our primitive ancestors who went around *au naturel* in the bright sunlight. It is known that bones of well-nourished animals become more densely mineralized as they grow older. Any doctor who specializes in X-rays has seen human bones that have become extremely thin in old age. Since your body can store large amounts of calcium in your bones, and since it is known that these deposits are heavily drawn upon in old age, it would seem in harmony with an intelligent program of nutrition to maintain a vitamin D intake that will promote the absorption and storage of calcium and phosphorus during the adult years.

If you choose to follow the recommendation of the National Research Council, you can easily achieve this by the use of one quart of vitamin D enriched milk per day—skim milk if you favor your arteries. If you wish to have a higher intake of this vitamin, you will probably need to go in for sun bathing or use a vitamin D capsule or tablet. For myself, I maintain a vitamin

6. *Recommended Dietary Allowances, Revised 1958,* Publication 589, p. 17. (Washington, D.C.: National Academy of Sciences—National Research Council, 1958.)

D intake of 1,000 units per day. Since your body can store large amounts of this vitamin, it is not necessary to take it daily. You may wish to choose a high-potency capsule that will be taken every week or every other week.

VITAMIN E (TOCOPHERALS)

Vitamin E is probably the most controversial vitamin. Research has proved that it is essential to the fertility of both male and female rats. To characterize this vitamin as essential to reproduction, the term "tocopheral" was coined from the Greek words *tokos* (childbirth) and *phero* (I bring). It has been found that rats and other animals deficient in vitamin E develop a paralysis similar to muscular dystrophy in humans. It has also been found that the lack of vitamin E leads to heart abnormalities and death in many animals. Scientific attempts to show that vitamin E prevents or cures similar problems with humans have not been successful.[7]

Dr. Edward S. Gordon of the University of Wisconsin has stated, "It is very obvious, therefore, that the sum total of our knowledge of vitamin E at the present time is woefully incomplete. Evidence from animal experiments leads to the almost inescapable conclusion that this vitamin plays some vital role in human nutrition as well. Elucidation of that function stands as a challenging problem for the future." [8] *It is interesting to note that human milk contains more vitamin E than cow's milk.*

Vitamin E is known to have several important functions in our bodies. It will help keep vitamin A from being destroyed and thus assist you in building

7. *Nutrition Reviews*, Vol. 18, p. 228, 1960.
8. Edgar S. Gordon, "Pyridoxine, Pantothenic Acid, Biotin, Inositol, and Vitamin E," from Jolliffe, *et al., op. cit.,* p. 618.

up large stores of vitamin A in your liver. It plays a part in many complex chemical reactions in your body. It has been found that when you follow a diet rich in linoleic acid and other unsaturated fats, your need for vitamin E is increased. Unlike vitamins A and D, large amounts are not toxic.

SOURCES OF VITAMIN E

Vitamin E is present in small quantities in many foods. The richest sources are vegetable oils such as corn oil, cottonseed oil, and particularly soybean and wheat germ oil. Other than oils, wheat germ, soybeans, and rice bran are the best sources. Most other foods contain relatively small amounts. An egg contains one and a half milligrams. You can eat your way through three and a half ounces of lettuce and only get one-half a milligram.

Here's the way some foods stack up on vitamin E: [9]

Food	Milligrams
Olive oil, 1 tbs.	1
Turnip greens, 3½ oz.	2
Peanut oil, refined, 1 tbs.	3
Peanut butter, 1 tbs.	3
Sweet potatoes, 3½ oz.	4
Sardines, 3½ oz.	5
Peas, 3½ oz.	6
French dressing, 1 tbs.	6
Fish roe, 3½ oz.	6
Kale, 3½ oz.	8

9. Compiled from: F. Bicknell and F. Prescott, *The Vitamins in Medicine*, pp. 629-631. (New York: Grune and Stratton, 1953.) P. L. Harris, M. L. Quaife, and W. J. Swanson, "Vitamin E Content of Foods," *Journal of Nutrition*, Vol. 40, pp. 367-381, 1950. Data on Compositions of Food Products of Best Foods Division, Corn Products Company. (Corn Products Institute of Nutrition, Argo, Illinois, March 1961.)

Food	Milligrams
Italian dressing, 1 tbs.	8
Peanuts, 3½ oz.	9
Corn oil, 1 tbs.	10
Margarine (Mazola type), 1 tbs.	10
Mayonnaise, commercial, 1 tbs.	10
Cottonseed oil, refined, 1 tbs.	13
Soybeans, 3½ oz.	19
Soybean oil, refined, 1 tbs.	20
Wheat germ, 3½ oz.	27
Wheat germ oil, 1 tbs.	36

WORKING TOWARD OPTIMAL LEVELS OF VITAMIN E

The National Research Council has not formulated allowances for vitamin E. Reasoning from the known facts of various animal experiments, Drs. Hickman and Harris estimated the needs of healthy adults for vitamin E to be about 30 milligrams daily. Analysis has shown an average vitamin E content of good diets to be about half this much. This apparently leaves the average American with a shortage of around 15 milligrams daily. This should be no problem for you. If you are beginning to achieve the levels of fat explained in Chapters 6 and 7, your intake of vitamin E through unsaturated vegetable oils will probably provide you with the suggested 30 milligrams daily. If in addition to vegetable oils containing vitamin E, you use a half-cup of wheat germ per day, you will pick up another 16 milligrams. Unlike the other oil-soluble vitamins, there is no known toxic level for vitamin E.

VITAMIN K

Vitamin K takes care of itself with very little special attention on our part. The story of vitamin K is short and simple. Research thus far indicates that it has one main function—to enable your blood to clot. If you had no vitamin K, you could bleed to death from a small wound. Doctors may prescribe it with surgery or childbirth to control bleeding.

Vitamin K is richly supplied by green leafy vegetables, egg yolks, soybean oil, and liver. Even if your diet is deficient in this vitamin, there is general agreement that beneficial types of intestinal bacilli will probably make an adequate supply for you. Like other oil-soluble vitamins, it is not damaged by the usual cooking methods. Since your approach to optimal nutrition will automatically lead you to foods rich in this vitamin, you can just relax—vitamin K-wise.

Chapter 15

BENEFITS OF CALCIUM AND PHOSPHOROUS

"One of the most likely uses of atomic energy," said O. D. Flynn, "seems to be the cooking of the world's goose." In the arms race between the United States and Russia, both sides have exploded large atomic bombs that sent trillions upon trillions of particles of strontium 90 into the upper atmosphere. Fast-moving winds have scattered this radioactive element over the entire earth. Strontium 90 was first detected in animal bones, dairy products, and soil in 1953. It is now in the bodies of all human beings regardless of their age or where they live.

When strontium 90 is absorbed into your body from food, it is deposited in your bones. High concentrations of it can cause bone cancer and possibly leukemia—a cancer of the bone marrow that interferes with the production of red blood cells. The amounts that have been absorbed by human beings thus far are thought to be below harmful limits.

Strontium 90 is present in every mouthful of food you eat. Plants absorb this radioactive material from the soil. Animals eat the plants, and human beings eat both plants and animals and their products—milk, meat, and eggs. It has been found that when animals are fed diets high in calcium, their bodies absorb less radioactive strontium than those with diets low in calcium. In one experiment, the rats on a diet rich in calcium absorbed only about one-fourth as much strontium as those with lower amounts of calcium. Similar results were obtained in experiments with cows. The United States Department of Agriculture has warned us, "If people react in the same way, it will be important to have high intakes and body reserves of calcium as built-in protection against radioactivity." [1]

Children growing up in this atomic age have about six to eight times more strontium 90 in their bones than their parents. I am sure future generations will wonder about the megaton madness that makes it necessary to contaminate the food supply with radioactive fallout. In the meantime, diets containing generous amounts of calcium as well as other nutrients will offer you and me the best protection we can get. It has been found that careful washing may remove as much as 60 per cent of the strontium 90 content of vegetables.[2]

ADDED LONGEVITY THROUGH CALCIUM

You will recall from Chapter 1 that Dr. Sherman's rats fed on Diet B had greater vitality and longevity than the rats on Diet A with less milk. Since the doubling of the milk in Diet B increased the vitamin A and B_2 intake as well as that of calcium, Dr. Sherman made further experiments to find out whether the increase of calcium alone in Diet A would give added health benefits. When he increased the calcium in Diet A by 75

1. *Food, The Yearbook of Agriculture 1959*, p. 118. (Department of Agriculture, Washington, D.C.: U.S. Government Printing Office.)
2. *Bulletin of the Atomic Scientists*, Vol. XVII, No. 3, p. 44, March 1962.

per cent without making any changes in the amounts of other nutrients, he found the following evidences of higher health:

1. More rapid growth.
2. The female was able to bear young earlier.
3. Females had a longer reproductive life.
4. They were able to bear more young.
5. Of the young born, more reached maturity.
6. The length of life for both males and females was increased.

Dr. Sherman found that when calcium alone was added to Diet A so as to make its calcium content the same as Diet B, the females showed improved breeding records. However, their average length of life was not as significantly increased as with males on the same food. This created a problem. Did it mean that the gals could not profit from the extra calcium? Could it be that they had invested their calcium in more and better offspring? Dr. Sherman made additional experiments. He found that unmated females with extra calcium gained as much in longevity as the males. He then made experiments to find what could be done to give added life to the females who were so busy producing young. He discovered that when they were given further increases in calcium, they were able to have a high reproduction rate and also enjoyed a longer life themselves!

When Dr. Sherman experimentally arrived at a presumably optimal level of calcium for both males and females, he found that the length of life of males was increased 11.5 per cent. Females lived 13.8 per cent longer! Dr. Sherman has pointed out that if these results apply to human nutrition (and no one knows for sure), the use of optimal calcium might extend human adult life by a similar percentage.

CALCIUM IS NEEDED FOR STRONG BONES

Our bones are not static structures like a piece of steel. They are living tissues that change slightly every day. There is an exchange of approximately 1 per cent of your calcium every 20 days. If the calcium which is constantly being removed from your bones is not replaced, they will gradually become thinner and thinner. Calcium-poor bones are weak and break much more easily than those densely saturated with this important mineral. The brittle and thin bones of older people are difficult to treat when they break. Healing may be slow and they may be too weak to hold pins.

Dr. Millicent L. Hathaway and Dr. Ruth M. Leverton have observed, "Height may be reduced as much as two inches because of fractures of the vertebrae, which are caused by pressure and result in rounding of the back. Such fractures may occur with relatively minor jolts or twists of the body and may not be recognized at the time they happen." [3] With liberal amounts of calcium and vitamin D to build strong bones, plus ample vitamin C for connective tissue formation, you can build a strong spinal column that should not be subject to the excruciating pain of slipped or crushed discs.

When your diet furnishes liberal amounts of calcium, you can store this mineral inside the ends of your bones. This stored calcium will form crystal-like honeycombs that add greatly to the strength of the bone as well as provide a large reservoir of calcium for use by your body. It has been estimated that one ounce of bone-forming material when deposited in tiny crystals in bones will have a surface area of four million square inches! [4]

3. *Food, The Yearbook of Agriculture 1959, op. cit.,* p. 114.
4. *Ibid.,* p. 43.

Storage of Calcium in Ends of Bones

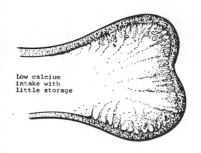
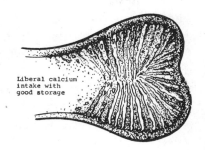

Low calcium
intake with
little storage

Liberal calcium
intake with
good storage

Blood circulates through these calcium storage areas. If your calcium intake for the day is below requirements, it will be immediately taken from the ends of your bones. If you go for a long time without adequate calcium in your diet, your calcium reservoir will be depleted and the bones themselves will be gradually thinned to provide your blood stream with the calcium it needs. The spinal and pelvic bones will usually be drawn on first. Hence the broken hips and ailing spines of many older people.

CALCIUM HAS MANY IMPORTANT USES THROUGHOUT THE BODY

Drs. Hathaway and Leverton in *Food, The Yearbook of Agriculture 1959* advised us, "A body well nourished with calcium and other nutrients can be expected to have good bone growth and development, a well-functioning nervous system, a high level of vigor and positive health at every age, and a longer period in the prime of life."

Although calcium is usually thought of in connection with bone formation, it also has many other vital uses that help you build optimal health. It interacts with other nutrients to help them do their job. It is needed, for example, with vitamin K to assist in the clotting of blood when there is a wound. It is used with vitamin C in the formation of collagen or intercellular cement that holds your body together. It assists in maintaining normal cell permeability, which enables your cells to select proper amounts of nutrients from the blood.

If the calcium level of your blood is low, your nerves may become easily stimulated and irritable. Your disposition may be grouchy and the effect of pain may be magnified. Perhaps added calcium might decrease the need for tranquilizers. Calcium regulates the action of muscles. When blood calcium is low, cramps or severe twitchings may occur. Calcium helps allay fatigue, probably by increasing the oxygen content of the muscle. The right proportion of calcium in the blood assists in maintaining the normal rhythmic contraction and relaxation of the heart. According to Dr. Sherman, calcium may also serve as a general regulator to protect the body from strains or stresses which may be thrown upon it by various dietary imbalances. Calcium also helps you keep your body firm and youthful.[5]

NEEDS DURING GROWTH

The bow legs, malformed chests, large foreheads, and slouched figures of so many people around us testify to the deficiency of this important mineral during growth. Calcium and phosphorus are needed in large quantities to enable a child to develop a strong body. Babies are born with flexible bones—possibly to make birth easier. Bones grow by depositing calcium and phosphorus on the outside surface while at the same time absorbing them from the inside. This hollows out the inside of the bone, and your skeleton is thus able

5. L. V. Heilbrunn, *The Scientific American*, June, 1951, pp. 60-63.

to grow and maintain strength without unnecessary weight. If bones grew only by adding material to the outside without simultaneously subtracting it from the inside, your skeleton would weigh so much that your muscles would have difficulty moving it around.

Teeth are formed both before birth and during infancy. If calcium is deficient during this period, narrow jaws will be formed that lack sufficient room for the growing teeth. This results in overcrowded, twisted teeth. They may also be more subject to decay in later life. Liberal amounts of milk and vitamin D each day during childhood may save hundreds of dollars in expensive and uncomfortable dental work later.

CALCIUM NEEDS IN OLD AGE

"Physicians have recently been commenting on the frequency with which X-ray photographs show rarefied [thinner] bones in older adults," Dr. L. Jean Bogert observed, "and they speculate on whether this may not be indicative of a life-long habit of taking less than 'optimum' amounts of these mineral elements in the diet." [6] Dr. W. M. Cobb has pointed out that there may be a gradual increase in the weight of your skeleton up to age thirty-five. It will then gradually decrease until you are sixty. After this age, your skeleton tends to lose calcium very rapidly.[7] Elderly people seem to assimilate calcium less efficiently and must have higher intakes if they are to maintain their calcium stores.

As we grow older, we should make a special effort to keep our diet rich in this important nutrient. Dr. McCay of Cornell observed, ". . . the ability of old rats to select diets adequate in calcium seems to decline as age advances. In early life the young rat has the ability

6. L. Jean Bogert, *Nutrition and Physical Fitness*, 7th ed., pp. 148-149. (Philadelphia: W. B. Saunders Company, 1954.)
7. W. M. Cobb, in A. I. Lansing, ed., *Problems of Ageing*, 3rd ed. (Baltimore: Williams and Wilkins Co., 1952.)

to select a diet containing calcium. . . . In old age the rat becomes an 'old fool' and will die while drinking a 10 per cent sugar solution to satisfy its taste rather than eating a diet to meet its nutritional requirements. Thus in old age when the body's need for calcium in the diet increases, the ability to select this diet seems to disappear." [8]

If your diet is not sufficiently rich in calcium to enable you to maintain the calcium content of your bones, they will become thinner and thinner as you grow older. A fracture may not heal well, and even metal pins may be of little use. Dallas and Nordin have pointed out that a slight calcium deficiency over ten or twenty years may destroy 30 per cent of your skeleton and give you a painful condition known as "osteoporosis." [9]

MILK IS THE MAIN SOURCE OF CALCIUM

You have probably found by studying the Food Table that without a fairly liberal use of milk and its products, it is almost impossible to have an adequate calcium intake. One quart of milk or buttermilk per day supplies 144 per cent of the recommended allowance. Many mothers add a heaping tablespoon of powdered skim milk to each glass of regular milk. This "fortified" milk adds to their children's intake of protein, vitamins and minerals. Milk products such as cottage cheese and yogurt are helpful in meeting your calcium needs. Leafy vegetables such as turnip greens provide fair amounts. Meats contain little calcium. Seafoods such as sardines are an exception since the soft bones are eaten. Some shellfish such as oysters and

8. Clive M. McCay, "Diet and Aging," *Vitamins and Hormones,* Vol. 7, p. 154, 1949.

9. I. Dallas and B. E. C. Nordin, "The Relation Between Calcium Intake and Roentgenologic Osteoporosis," *American Journal of Clinical Nutrition,* Vol. II, p. 263, 1962.

shrimp contain a worthwhile amount of calcium. Most other foods provide only small amounts.

If you are one of those who think milk is for children only, or if you are allergic to it, or if you don't like milk, you have my deepest sympathy. Your journey toward optimal nutrition will be difficult indeed without a generous intake of milk. Milk is not only the main source of calcium, but it is also an excellent source of protein and vitamin B_2 in addition to containing many other vitamins and minerals that are needed by your body.

Tests have shown that the cow's body helps to screen out radioactive strontium 90. The meat of the cow, for example, only contains one-fourth of the strontium 90 that is found in the fodder. When you drink the milk, however, you are only getting one-tenth as much as in the original fodder! [10] *Thus, swallow for swallow, milk is less contaminated with strontium 90 than almost any other food you can eat except fish.*

Scientists have studied the usefulness of various types of milk. They found that there was no appreciable difference in the nutritive value of liquid whole milk, liquid skim milk, pasteurized milk, homogenized milk, evaporated milk, or dried milk solids. To determine if the growth of children was influenced by the kind of milk they drink, the U.S. Public Health Service kept records of the weight and height of 3,700 children between ten months and six years old. They found that those who used pasteurized milk gained slightly more in height and weight, but they did not consider the difference significant. There was a slightly higher incidence of infection-borne diseases among the children that had raw milk.

As long as your heart beats, you have a continuous

10. *Food, The Yearbook of Agriculture 1959*, p. 118. (Department of Agriculture, Washington, D.C.: U.S. Government Printing Office.)

need for the nutrients that milk supplies. Children and adults who do not have at least one quart of milk per day are handicapped in their quest for optimal nutrition. For people who are allergic to milk, it is suggested they make every effort to find some form of milk that is acceptable—perhaps buttermilk, milk powder, or yogurt may be used. An attempt should be made to put larger and larger quantities of dried skim milk powder into soups, mashed potatoes, casseroles, breads, and other dishes.

If it is impossible to use milk in any form, bone powder can be used to provide calcium. A level teaspoon of bone powder contains approximately the recommended daily calcium allowance. This amount can easily be stirred into foods. Be sure to use bone powder with the texture of talcum powder. The coarser bone meal is not as easily assimilated by your body. Like vitamin C, more will be absorbed if it is not taken all at one time but distributed throughout the day. Sometimes physicians recommend calcium gluconate or calcium lactate tablets. A one-gram tablet supplies 125 per cent of the daily recommended allowance.

CALCIUM NOT AVAILABLE IN SOME FOODS

The green leaves of plants are one of the best sources of calcium after milk or milk products. However, oxalic acid in the leaves of chard, beet greens, rhubarb, and spinach prevents the absorption of calcium. You will note in our Food Table that although calcium is present in these leaves, it has been assigned a value of 0 per cent since it cannot be used by your body. Experiments have shown, however, that the oxalic acid in these foods will not prevent the absorption of calcium from other foods that are eaten at the same time.

Cocoa and chocolate contain oxalic acid, and at one time nutritionists were concerned whether or not chocolate milk was well absorbed. It has been found, however, that the calcium in chocolate milk is absorbed satisfactorily. The oxalic acid tends only to bind the small amount of calcium in the chocolate.

Soaking or cooking in water will cause calcium and phosphorus to dissolve. Cabbage boiled ten minutes loses 23 per cent of its calcium and 20 per cent of the phosphorus. These nutrients are not lost if the cooking water is utilized in some form. Vegetables that are steamed or baked retain their minerals.

FOR MAXIMUM ABSORPTION

A deficiency of hydrochloric acid in your stomach will affect calcium absorption. This acid assists in dissolving calcium so that the calcium will enter your blood stream. Dr. A. C. Ivy found that 23 per cent of the people over sixty are deficient in this vital digestive fluid.[11] If tests show that your output of hydrochloric acid is deficient, your doctor may prescribe hydrochloric acid tablets to be taken at mealtime. It has also been found that the use of laxatives, which hurry the food through the intestines, will lower the absorption of calcium.

You will recall from Chapter 14 that vitamin D is essential for the absorption of calcium. If this vitamin is not available, little or no calcium will be absorbed into your blood stream even though your diet may be rich in this mineral. It has also been found that when calcium-rich foods are eaten at a meal containing either orange juice or protein, the calcium is absorbed more efficiently.

A small amount of fat helps a calcium-rich food enter the blood stream from the intestines. To get the greatest calcium benefits from skim milk, it is helpful to take it with a meal containing fat or oil. The "Total

11. A. C. Ivy in E. V. Cowdry, ed., *Problems of Ageing*. (Baltimore: Williams and Wilkins Co., 1942.)

Fat" column in the Food Table will indicate what
foods contain fat. It has been found, however, that
when too much fat is eaten with a meal, a calcium soap
is formed that is not absorbed. Thus, calcium in your
diet will be wasted if it is accompanied by too little
or too much fat.

It has been found that humans only absorb about
20 per cent to 30 per cent of their calcium intake. The
rest is eliminated with food waste. If you absorb more
calcium into your blood than your body needs, it is
readily excreted by the kidneys. Thus excessive amounts
of calcium are not toxic.

WORKING TOWARD OPTIMAL CALCIUM IN YOUR DIET

The human body is remarkable in its ability to
adapt to many different levels of calcium. In some
countries where people have a low amount of calcium in
their diet, they manage to avoid signs of calcium deficiency with a daily total of about 38 per cent to 50
per cent. Such an intake seems far from optimal.

The stress of pregnancy requires large amounts of
calcium. If necessary, this mineral will be taken from
the mother's bones to provide for the baby if adequate
calcium is not available in her diet. If the mother's
nutrition or health will not permit the production of
good-quality milk, the milk flow will decrease or stop.
The National Research Council recommends that a
mother increase her calcium intake to 188 per cent during the second half of pregnancy. When nursing, even
more is required. They suggest at this time a calcium
total of 250 per cent. For a child of one to three years
they recommend a calcium total of 125 per cent. From
the tenth to twelfth year, calcium should be increased
to 150 per cent and teenage boys should get 175 per
cent.

Scientists have found that a daily calcium total

of 125 per cent in elderly men prevented calcium loss, and in some men permitted a small storage of this valuable mineral. Dr. Sherman has stated, ". . . wherever, within normal bounds, we have a choice of higher or lower calcium intake levels, the choice of the more liberal consumption of calcium may confidently be expected to contribute more both to immediate efficiency and to the higher health of the long run of the life cycle." [12]

Research by Drs. Henry and Kon indicated that rats who became accustomed to a very high intake of calcium had more difficulty retaining calcium in their bones than those accustomed to a lower intake. This occurred especially in old age.[13] Since this may apply to humans, it would seem that optimal calcium means *not too little and not too much.*

Your diet should be sufficiently rich in calcium to allow you to store large amounts of this mineral in your bones. The reserve may be vital during your later years when the absorption of calcium from your diet becomes difficult. Dr. Sherman has recommended a daily calcium total of 125 per cent for men and women. Perhaps with radioactivity increasing all around us, twice this amount of calcium may help our bodies fight off the effects of radioactive strontium 90. It seems likely that future research may indicate that once the age of sixty is reached, the amount of calcium in the diet should be gradually increased by several per cent each year.

THE ROLE OF PHOSPHORUS

Phosphorus also plays a part in building bones. It is one of the most active minerals in your body, as it

12. Henry C. Sherman, "Calcium in the Chemistry of Food and Nutrition," *Nutrition Reviews*, Vol. 10, p. 99, 1952.
13. Henry and Kon, *British Journal of Nutrition*, Vol. 7, p. 147, 1953.

forms a part of every cell. It is important in regulating many internal activities of your body and it interacts with other nutrients to enable them to do their work. Phosphorus plays an essential part in cell reproduction. When it is inadequately supplied, your body will dissolve some bone to meet the day-to-day phosphorus needs of your tissues. Many B vitamins are effective only when combined with phosphorus. Carbohydrates and fats cannot be used for energy by the body unless this mineral is available. Phosphorus also assists in maintaining the normal acid-base balance of the blood.

Fortunately, phosphorus is no problem in your diet. Nutritionists have a working rule: "Take care of the calcium and the phosphorus will take care of itself." It is present in most foods and is especially concentrated in those containing protein and iron. When you work toward an optimal intake of protein, iron, and calcium, you will probably have a near-optimal amount of phosphorus.

In experiments with rats, it was found that calcium and phosphorus should approximately balance each other in the body. An excessive amount of phosphorus will lower the absorption of calcium—especially if vitamin D is deficient. This led to the formulation of a calcium-phosphorus ratio. Most nutritionists try to balance diets so that the amount of phosphorus is either equal to the amount of calcium or does not exceed calcium by over 50 per cent. Recent experiments seem to indicate that this calcium-phosphorus ratio is not as important for humans as for rats. If you supply your body with a generous amount of calcium and have an adequate amount of protein (which is a good source of phosphorus), you may be sure that these two minerals will be adequately balanced in your body.

Chapter 16

IRON BUILDS RED BLOOD

If you are optimally nourished, your blood will probably contain a generous mixture of proteins, vitamins, minerals, sugars, and small amounts of the proper kinds of fat. Also floating around in your blood are about 25 billion red blood cells that act as "redcaps" to carry oxygen to the 26 trillion cells throughout your body. These blood cells are so small that it takes 3,200 in single file to measure an inch. They absorb oxygen as they travel through the lungs, and feed this oxygen to the ever-hungry cells of your body. When these tiny discs pick up a load of oxygen in the lungs, they are bright red in color. They lose this color and become blue after they deliver their oxygen to the cells.

Iron is the mineral that enables your red blood cells to alternately absorb oxygen in the lungs and release it to the cells throughout your body. A little over half of your iron is concentrated in your blood. If you are deficient, the oxygen-carrying capacity of your blood is lowered. Your ears may be paler and your nails may lack the pink glow of health. You will gradually feel weaker, your breath will be short, your appetite will be poor, you may have headaches, and there will be a general slowing up of the vital functions of your body. Other symptoms of iron-deficiency anemia are sore tongue, capricious appetite, flatulence, constipation, and brittle ridged fingernails.

Red blood cells are made in the marrow of the large bones in your body. These busy little porters have a life span of about 120 days. Your body's efficiency in conserving iron is remarkable. When they are worn out they are retired by the spleen and the precious iron they contain is reprocessed so that about 90 per cent of it can be reused by your body. When you have a good supply of red blood cells, there will be about five million of them in only twelve drops of blood.

The most common type of anemia is due to a lack of iron. Although an anemic person tends to be pale, such appearances cannot always be relied on since the pigmentation of the skin can be misleading. Doctors can determine iron-deficiency anemia simply by comparing the red color of the blood with a standard color scale. A deep red color indicates adequate iron. The paler the blood, the more severe the anemia. Another type of anemia may result if the diet is deficient in folic acid. Still another type, pernicious anemia, is caused by a failure to absorb vitamin B_{12}.

HEAVY NEEDS FOR IRON

Before birth, a baby accumulates an extra store of iron in his liver. Since milk is low in iron, this must last through the nursing period. Even though the mother may be anemic, the infant generously helps himself from her low supply. Before the end of the nursing period, most infants today are given iron-rich foods such as egg yolk, chopped green vegetables, and meat to supplement their dwindling supply of iron. Their need is quite high because blood volume is increasing rapidly and large quantities of red blood cells must be produced. Dr. Mackey made a study of infants in London and found that 42 per cent of the breast-fed and 70 per cent of the bottle-fed infants were anemic. These infants were twice as susceptible to infection as those that had an adequate supply of iron in their diet. Throughout childhood and the teen years, large amounts of iron are needed to permit proper growth.

Iron is found in all living cells and it plays a fundamental role in their ceaseless change and growth. Women require more iron than men because they are subject to three losses unknown to men: menstruation, gestation, and lactation. Men sometimes even things out by developing a bleeding peptic ulcer, which can result in considerable blood loss.

The generous habit of donating blood can result in a loss that must be made up by added iron in the diet. An extra 60 per cent in your daily iron total for each transfusion per year will probably make up for this iron loss. This added iron must be continued for a whole year. Thus if you donate blood three times per year, add 180 per cent to your daily iron total to make up for it.[1]

IRON IS POORLY ABSORBED

An oversupply of water-soluble minerals such as calcium or phosphorus is rapidly excreted in the urine. The kidneys, however, cannot excrete iron. Your body's defense against an excessive iron intake lies in controlling the amount it absorbs. You usually only absorb from 5 per cent to 10 per cent of the iron in your

1. Carl V. Moore, "Iron and the Essential Trace Elements," from Michael G. Wohl and Robert S. Goodhart, eds., *Modern Nutrition in Health and Disease*, 2nd ed., p. 245. (Philadelphia: Lea and Febiger, 1960.) (The suggested 60 per cent addition to the daily iron total that appears above is based on Moore's figures with an assumed 10 per cent absorption efficiency.)

diet. If you are deficient in iron, your body may absorb a higher percentage.

It has been found that certain forms of iron are more readily used by the body than others. The iron in liver is well absorbed, but that in muscle meats is not well utilized. Vitamin C, when eaten with iron-rich meals, will add to the body's ability to absorb iron. Protein and vitamin E have a similar effect. The best sources of iron are foods rich in protein and B vitamins. They include organ meats such as liver and kidney, wheat germ, and yeast. Eggs, lean meats, beans, nuts, dried fruits, whole grains or enriched cereal foods, and all green leafy vegetables add substantially to the daily iron total.

Iron may be lost when food is carelessly prepared. When lima beans are boiled in a small amount of water, they will lose about 7 per cent of their iron. When they are boiled in a large amount of water, the loss will be about 25 per cent. When green cabbage is boiled ten minutes, it will lose about 16 per cent of the iron; sixty minutes of boiling will remove about 36 per cent. This mineral will not be lost if the cooking water is used for soups or stews. When vegetables are steamed as described in Chapter 13, there is practically no loss of iron or other minerals.

"To eat is human," said Mark Twain, "to digest— divine." As with other nutrients, iron is best absorbed by a healthy, well-functioning digestive system. When food is hurried through, as with diarrhea, or when laxatives are used, there is not time enough for proper absorption of iron or other nutrients. However, when the movement of food through the intestines is sluggish, as with constipation, the iron gradually changes to an insoluble form that cannot be digested.

It is possible to get too much iron, but this is not very likely. The Bantus in Africa cook their food in soft iron pots which results in an iron intake of ten to twenty times the daily allowance, and this often results in illness. But nutritionists who have studied the Bantus have suggested that if their intake of phosphorus and vitamin B₆ were adequate, their bodies would probably be able to resist the effects of excess iron.[2] As with other nutrients, as long as you get your iron from natural foods and not from pills or rusty iron pots, you need have little concern about a toxic oversupply.

AN APPROACH TO OPTIMAL IRON

If your iron total comes to 100 per cent as computed from our Food Table, you will be getting the amount of iron that the National Research Council recommends for 25-year-old moderately active American males. They suggest that women, due to the heavy iron loss during the fertile period of their lives, should have an iron total of 120 per cent. Infants after weaning should have an iron total of 50 per cent, and after 6 months this should be increased to 70 per cent. As you will note in the Recommended Allowances for Various Groups on page 216, children require from 70 per cent to 120 per cent, depending on their age, while teenage boys and girls should have a total of 150 per cent. During pregnancy and lactation, the National Research Council recommends that the iron total be maintained at 150 per cent.

Dr. Sherman has recommended a daily iron total of 120 per cent. Such an allowance will provide normal males with a 50 per cent margin of safety above their minimum requirement. Although girls and women can avoid signs of iron deficiency on the recommended

2. Stanley Davidson, A. P. Meiklejohn, and R. Passmore, *Human Nutrition and Dietetics*, p. 182. (Baltimore: The Williams and Wilkins Company, 1959.)

allowance of 120 per cent, *they will not have the same amount of iron available for general use by the body as males receiving the recommended allowance of 100 per cent.* I don't feel the gals should be shortchanged like this. If women wish to be on an iron par with men, the iron lost in menstruation, gestation, and lactation must be approximately balanced by a higher intake. Since the absorption of iron is at best about 10 per cent efficient, it is necessary for a woman to have an *extra* iron intake ten times the average amount lost if she wants to balance out these losses. It is thus necessary for a woman during her reproductive years to maintain an iron intake that totals 150 per cent to 200 per cent if she is to have the same amount of iron available for bodily use and storage as a man with an iron total of 100 per cent.[3]

As with other nutrients, experimental work with humans has not been performed which scientifically defines optimal levels of iron. The best we can do at this time is to use the nutritional and medical data that is available and make estimates as to what may constitute optimal levels. It is unusual today for physicians or nutritionists to recommend an iron intake for women that compensates for menstrual losses. Practically all current recommendations leave them with a considerably lower iron supply available for general body uses than is recommended for men. It would seem, however, that a program designed to approach optimal nutrition should attempt to replace these large iron losses of women.

From the above, it is obvious that any woman who wishes to work toward a possibly optimal level of iron must concentrate on iron-rich foods to a much greater

3. These recommendations are based on the quantitative utilization of iron as discussed by Carl V. Moore in Goodhart, *et al.*, *op. cit.*, p. 242.

extent than is necessary for the men in her family. If a wife eats 2,000 calories of the same foods that her husband consumes at the 3,000-calorie level, she will only have two-thirds of the iron that her husband will get. It would thus seem important for women and growing children to have a diet that is unusually rich in food containing iron. An aside to the girls—it may be helpful to go through the Food Table and circle all of those foods that are unusually high in this vital mineral.

Chapter 17

MINERALS MAKE A DIFFERENCE

Imagine a speck of iodine so small that 150,000 are required to make an ounce. This tiny amount per day can make the difference between good health and bad health, a normal neck or a swollen goiterous neck—even between life and death. In ancient times, people learned there was an unknown magic in burned sponge and seaweed that cured goiter. This time-tested lore was submerged in the ignorance of the Dark Ages. Modern science has now unveiled iodine as the nutrient vital to the thyroid gland, which is located a little below your Adam's apple. This iodine-hungry gland grabs iodine from your blood so greedily that there is 10,000 times more iodine in your thyroid than in your blood stream.

Your thyroid gland produces a hormone known as thyroxine, which regulates the tempo of your energy production. Thyroxine is about two-thirds iodine. If you are low in thyroxine, you are low in spirit, low in energy, and usually complaining about low temperature when everyone else is comfortable. When your thyroid gland is functioning normally, adequate amounts of thyroxine are carried by the blood stream throughout your body where it plays its part in making you the energetic, vivacious, and happy person that you should be.

When iodine is deficient in the diet, the thyroid gland seeks to compensate by increasing its size. If the deficiency in iodine is severe and prolonged, the swelling may greatly disfigure the neck. Iodine-deficient mothers may have children that are pot-bellied, pudgy dwarfs with low intelligence and low energy. Such unfortunate children are known as "cretins." Cretinism does not occur if even a few millionths of a gram of iodine is present in the diet.

In 1917, Dr. David Marine and Dr. O. P. Kimball gave iodine to children in the public schools of Akron, Ohio. One group of children received small daily doses of sodium iodide over a period of two weeks; this was repeated in the following semester. Out of 2,190 children who were given iodine, only five showed any enlargement of the thyroid gland. Among 2,305 children not taking iodine, 495 showed an increased enlargement of the neck. This pioneering experiment proved that goiter could be prevented or cured by iodine.

SOURCES OF IODINE

Soils that are deficient in iodine are scattered throughout the world. In the United States the "goiter belt" extends from Oregon to the western part of Maine, and from Nevada to the western part of Virginia. Foods grown in many parts of this area cannot be relied on to prevent the heartbreaking tragedies that occur when iodine is deficient.

The sea is rich in iodine and saltwater fish are an excellent source of this mineral. Ground seaweed or kelp may be used to provide iodine as well as other minerals. Soils near the seacoast which have received the fine mist from the sea for thousands of years are well supplied with iodine. Foods grown on these soils may be counted upon to supply your body liberally with this essential mineral.

The simplest way for most people to get iodine is through iodized salt. This salt to which a small amount of iodine has been added is usually available at no extra charge. Iodized salt was first put on the market in 1924 and it has proven effective in preventing goiter whenever it has been consistently used. Because of this salt, the rate of goiter in Michigan school children has dropped from 38.6 per cent in 1924 to 1.4 per cent in 1952. Unfortunately, less than one-half of the table salt sold in this country is iodized. The use of this salt in goiter areas has brought about a decrease in deaths from cancer of the thyroid. Since iodized salt costs no more than regular salt, many nutritionists feel that only iodized salt should be sold in the markets.

If for some reason the above suggestions are not practical for you, your doctor can prescribe an inexpensive preparation known as Lugol's solution. A few drops once a week will supply your need for iodine.

TOWARD OPTIMAL IODINE

According to Dr. George Curtis and Dr. M. B. Fertman of Ohio State University, the probable optimal intake of iodine is about two hundred millionths of a gram per day for a 154-pound adult. Slightly more than this amount is furnished by one-half a level teaspoon of iodized salt per day (about one-tenth of an ounce). These doctors have pointed out, "To thrive and function at his best under the ever-increasing demands of modern effort and production each individual should have, among other important elements, an adequate supply of iodine. . . . The increased physical activity and emotional stress resultant from present world tensions put increased demands upon the human body. An optimal response to these demands cannot be maintained without a sufficient supply of iodine." [1]

YOUR BODY'S NEED FOR SALT

The history of man's use of salt trails back into antiquity. Cakes of salt have been used for money and our word "salary" goes back to the Latin word for salt—*sal*. Since salt was considered the same as wealth, taxes have been based on how much salt a man owned. It was frequently included in offerings to the gods.

Table salt is about 40 per cent sodium and 60 per cent chlorine—both of which are needed by your body. Chlorine is used to make hydrochloric acid that enables your stomach to digest protein. Sodium is an important mineral that must be present in the blood at all times.

Animals that live on grass which contains little natural sodium will travel long distances to a "salt lick." Carnivorous animals that eat meat do not need an outside source of salt. Nomadic tribes who use meat and drink milk (both of which contain sodium) usually do not require more sodium than is available in their food. Others living on cereals and vegetables low in sodium require extra salt—especially when they live in a hot climate. Groups living near the ocean may get sodium from the use of saltwater fish.

Your body's need for salt may soar if you are active in hot weather, for large amounts of sodium are lost when you perspire. Weakness or fainting may follow if you do not rapidly replenish the lost sodium. You have probably seen photos of military events in

1. George M. Curtis and M. Been Fertman, "Iodine Malnutrition," from Norman Jolliffe, F. F. Tisdall, and Paul R. Cannon, eds., *Clinical Nutrition*, p. 390. (New York: Hoeber Medical Division, Harper & Row, Publishers, Inc., 1950.)

which one of the soldiers has collapsed and is lying unconscious on the ground. A good salting of the food he ate for breakfast may have prevented this "heat-stroke." When men work in unusual heat (such as the boiler room of a ship), the lack of salt can be fatal if extra salt is not used to replace the rapid loss. When you are low in sodium, drinking large amounts of water may actually bring on heatstroke, because water will dilute salt in your blood.

A lack of adequate salt can bring on loss of energy, headache, giddiness, cramps, lack of appetite, and nausea. Only water plus salt when you are perspiring very heavily over a prolonged period will meet your body's needs. But don't use salt tablets habitually in the summer unless you are really doing some prolonged sweaty work.

The body may also be rapidly depleted of its reserve salt when high fever causes continuous sweating or when diarrhea is present. Deaths due to a lack of salt have occurred with babies suffering from diarrhea in the summertime.

SALT AND WEIGHT REDUCTION

Many reducing diets tell you not to use salt. For normal people, this can be misleading—if not fraudulent. Here's why. When you lower your salt intake, your body must excrete extra water to maintain the proper saline balance of your blood. *It is thus possible to lose several pounds of water by curtailing salt.* You will weigh a pound less for each pint of water you lose. This may make you feel good when you step on the scales, but it has nothing to do with getting rid of fat, which is what you're after. If you honestly want to know whether you're reducing, let your salt intake stay at its normal level. If your scale then has good news for you, you'll know that you've lost fat—not just water that will rapidly be regained when your diet returns to normal.

WORKING TOWARD OPTIMAL SALT

As with other nutrients, too much or too little is inadvisable. Doctors for many years have known that high blood pressure (hypertension) is sometimes helped by eliminating sodium from the diet. They have long suspected that *excessive salt* might sometimes play a part in the development of high blood pressure.[2] Recent studies of hypertension in Japan have confirmed that a high intake of salt is associated with the development of high blood pressure. For example, farmers in northern Honshu use about one ounce of salt per day, while those in the middle and southern part of Japan average about one-half ounce per day. The Honshu area, where salt is used the most liberally, has the greatest amount of high blood pressure and deaths from strokes. The average American male uses about one-third ounce of salt per day.[3]

An optimal diet as approached in this book will probably provide you with adequate sodium to meet your normal needs at normal temperatures without the use of added table salt. As mentioned in the previous section, about one-half level teaspoon of iodized salt per day will provide you with what may be an optimal level of iodine. If this amount is used on your food each day in addition to the sodium naturally present in your food, you should have plenty of this mineral to meet your normal needs. If you are exercising heavily in the summertime, or engaged in heavy, sweaty work, or suffering from diarrhea or fever, extra salt should be taken with each extra quart of water you drink.

2. *Journal of the American Medical Association*, Vol. 178, p. 865, November 25, 1961.
3. Lewis K. Dahl, "Salt, Fat and Hypertension: The Japanese Experience," *Nutrition Reviews*, Vol. 18, p. 99, 1960.

FLUORINE IS NECESSARY FOR DENTAL HEALTH

Around 1931 it was discovered that excessive fluorine in drinking water caused a discoloration of tooth enamel. Several cities changed their water supply so as to reduce the fluorine to a minimum. A few years later, the surprising discovery was made that children born after the water supply had been changed suffered more dental decay than those who had drunk the fluoridated water. Additional research showed that when water contains one part per million of fluorine, the children in that community will have from 25 per cent to 50 per cent fewer cavities than those in a community without the benefits of this amount of fluorine.

When fluorine is applied by dentists to the teeth of young children, decay may be reduced by as much as 25 per cent to 40 per cent. This requires a number of applications during the years when the teeth are developing. Since many parents may be forgetful, the American Dental Association and the American Medical Association recommended that fluorine be added to the water supply in areas that are low in this mineral.

As often happens when we tamper with our food, water and air, experience over a number of years may indicate drawbacks. Dr. John A. Yiamouyiannis and Dr. Dean Burk at the 65th Annual Meeting of the American Society of Biological Chemistry in San Francisco on June 10, 1977 pointed out that the mutagenic and tumor-inducing effects of fluoride that have been discovered in animal experiments may also affect human beings who drink artificially-fluoridated water. These scientists checked the cancer death rates of the ten largest cities fluoridated before 1957. They compared them with the cancer death rates of the ten largest non-fluoridated (as of 1969) cities with comparable average pre-fluoridation cancer death rates.[4]

After the water supply had been artificially fluoridated, the average cancer death rate of the ten cities using fluorine

[4]John A. Yiamouyiannis and Dean Burk. Biological Pharmacology. IV p. 1707).

increased by 15 to 20 percent by 1969 as compared to only 2 to 5 per cent in the non-fluoridated cities, according to these researchers. They also pointed out that the cancer death rate of fluoridated Providence increased 25 per cent compared to only 8 per cent in non-fluoridated Boston. The cancer death rate of fluoridated San Francisco rose 19 per cent compared to only 4 per cent in nearby non-fluoridated Oakland. Their research indicates that in the state of California, the 1970 death rate of artificially fluoridated communities with populations over 10,000 was 29 per cent higher than in the rest of the state. By projecting statistics, they estimated that a minimum of 20,000 to 30,000 excess cancer deaths per year occur in cities that are exposed to artificially fluoridated waters.

All of us who are interested in the best possible nutrition should do everything we can to try to create an environment where we can breathe the purest possible air, drink the purest possible water, and eat foods grown on rich soils and without toxic sprays.

WORKING TOWARD OPTIMAL MINERALS

Minerals are as important to you as proteins, vitamins, and fats. The chain of nutrition is no stronger than its weakest link. People lacking in nutritional know-how can easily be on a precarious balance with calcium, iron, iodine, sodium, and fluorine.[5] We have discussed these essential minerals in detail because *special care may be needed to avoid deficiencies.* You probably have been low in one or more of these minerals many times in your life.

In addition to the above mentioned minerals, your body also requires phosphorus, chlorine, potassium, magnesium, copper, cobalt, sulphur, manganese, molybdenum, selenium, and zinc. What a headache it would be if our supply of these were also on a touch-and-go basis! Fortunately, these minerals are abundantly sup-

5. "Bone Density and Fluoride Ingestion," *Nutrition Reviews,* Vol. 19, pp. 198-199, 1961.

plied by natural fruits, vegetables, meats, dairy products, and seafoods. If your diet meets the nutritional standards of this book, you will probably get generous quantities of the minerals listed in this paragraph. It is possible, however, that people on reducing diets or folks whose inactivity requires few calories may not get an adequate quantity of some of these minerals. This can probably be prevented by emphasizing foods with a high Vitamin-Mineral Index. Most of the minerals are concentrated in the liver of all animals. The liver, acting as the chemical workshop of the body, serves as a storage depot for these minerals used in regulating the body. Liver, kidneys, heart, and other organ meats are in general far higher in minerals than muscle meats such as steak.

In addition to the minerals we have mentioned so far, the following are frequently found in tiny amounts in the bodies of animals: aluminum, arsenic, barium, boron, bromine, caesium, chromium, lead, lithium, nickel, ribidium, silicon, silver, strontium, tellurium, tin, titanium, and vanadium—almost everything but the kitchen sink! It is not known whether these are essential to human nutrition.[6] If future research shows these trace minerals to be essential to human nutrition, the chances are that the road to optimal nutrition you are following will have supplied excellent amounts.

The National Research Council has indicated that antagonisms may occur between relatively small increases in trace minerals. They caution against their indiscriminate use in mineral pills or capsules.[7] Balance is important. In view of the small amount of knowledge

6. Carl V. Moore, "Iron and the Essential Trace Elements," from Michael G. Wohl, Robert S. Goodhart, eds., *Modern Nutrition in Health and Disease*, 2nd ed., p. 235. (Philadelphia: Lea and Febiger, 1960.)

7. *Recommended Dietary Allowances, Revised 1958*, Publication 589, p. 22. (Washington, D.C.: National Academy of Sciences—National Research Council.)

that we have at this time about trace minerals in optimal human nutrition, it is generally best to rely on natural foods for these nutrients.

TOP–QUALITY SOIL

Optimal health has its roots in optimal soil. It is important to remember that if minerals are not present in soil, they will not be in plants grown in the soil. In working toward optimal nutrition, you must insist on quality produce. Carrots should be a deep orange in color—not just enclosed in tinted bags that give a beautiful appearance. Cracked and split vegetables, unevenly ripened ones, and those with other signs of plant disease were probably grown on poor soils deficient in minerals. Healthy plants cannot be grown in deficient soil, and you and I cannot achieve the highest level of health without the important minerals that nature offers us in healthy plants grown in well-balanced soils.

Chapter 18

FIGHTING DISEASE BY BUILDING HEALTH

"If I had my way," said Robert Ingersoll, "I would be catching health instead of disease." In a discussion with the head of a clinic, I once asked, "Would your patients benefit by building up their health through improved nutrition? Would medicine work more successfully if your patients were optimally nourished?"

"Yes," he replied, "but if I tried it, my patients would leave me. They come to me wanting a quick miracle pulled out of my black bag. Some of my patients tell *me* what to prescribe for *them!* They insist on injections of penicillin and other 'wonder' drugs, even if I tell them an antibiotic is not helpful for their condition. When I don't give them what they want, they simply go to the doctor who will."

Another doctor once told me that he had given up trying to help people nutritionally. He said that most of his patients responded to his attempts to get them to improve their diet as though he were trying to change their religion! They want to eat what they want to eat! If they get some ailment, they expect him to cure it pronto by pills and shots. This neglect of nutrition is most unfortunate, for as the *Journal of Clinical Nu-*

trition has pointed out, ". . . all physicians are involved with nutrition, for it is not the disease that is important, but the person who has the disease—and each person is the product of his nutrition." [1]

Dr. Herbert Ratner, Associate Clinical Professor of Preventive Medicine and Public Health at the Stritch School of Medicine, Loyola University, has commented on a paradox regarding our health: ". . . we are the wealthiest country in the world—yet one of the unhealthiest countries in the world. Dr. Paul Dudley White, President Eisenhower's physician, has made the allegation of unhealthiness on numerous occasions. I would agree with him about our low-level wellness in America. We are flabby, overweight, and have a lot of dental caries, fluoridation notwithstanding. Our gastrointestinal system operates like a sputtering gas engine. We can't sleep; we can't get going when we are awake. We have neuroses; we have high blood pressure. Neither our hearts nor our heads last as long as they should. Coronary disease at the peak of life has hit epidemic proportions. Suicide is one of the leading causes of death (fourth between the ages of 15 and 44). We suffer from a plethora of the diseases of civilization." [2]

In this chapter we will review the work of Dr. Robert McCarrison, who was knighted by the British Crown for his outstanding work in nutrition. Dr. E. V. McCollum, Professor of Biochemistry at Johns Hopkins University, said of him, "Intellectual honesty, enthusiasm, curiosity, studious attention to interpreting his observations in the full light of the work of others, courage of conviction in unusual measure in defending

1. Editorial: "What is Nutrition?" *Journal of Clinical Nutrition*, No. 1, p. 149, 1953.
2. Herbert Ratner, *Medicine*, an interview by Donald McDonald. One of a Series of Interviews on the American Character. (Santa Barbara, California: Center for the Study of Democratic Institutions, 1962.)

his considered conclusions are characteristic of him. He possessed not only knowledge but wisdom." [3]

In the early part of this century, young Dr. McCarrison was stationed by the British government in the mountains of northern India (now Pakistan). He noticed that certain groups possessed unusually high levels of health. It had been reported that among some folks in northern India, coronary heart disease, arthritis, diabetes, polio, and cancer were almost unknown! Some of these people had such remarkable physical endurance that they could travel on foot for one hundred miles without stopping for sleep. How did they get this unusual health and energy? Was it heredity? Was it the environment in which they lived? Was their food responsible? Dr. McCarrison's inquiring mind wanted scientific answers to these questions.

EXPERIMENTS WITH HUMAN DIET

When he became director of the government laboratory at Coonoor, India, Dr. McCarrison began an experiment in which he raised 1,189 white rats on a diet similar to that eaten by the unusually vigorous people of northern India. Most of these rats were maintained for a period corresponding to about fifty years in a human life. They were then sacrificed and Dr. McCarrison autopsied each one. During the two and a quarter years of this experiment, Dr. McCarrison found no case of illness! In his laborious post-mortem examination of 1,189 white rats, he found no evidence of disease other than an occasional tapeworm cyst. "Disease and death have been excluded, almost completely . . . ," he was able to report. [4]

3. E. V. McCollum, "Sir Robert McCarrison's Place in the History of Nutritional Research," from H. M. Sinclair, ed., *The Work of Sir Robert McCarrison*, p. xxxv. (London: Faber and Faber Limited, 1953.)

4. *Ibid.*, p. 285.

Most of the people in India fail to achieve the high level of health that inspired Dr. McCarrison's experiment. To further explore the relationship between nutrition and health, Dr. McCarrison fed 2,243 white rats the faulty diets of other Indian groups which lacked in health and vigor. When he personally autopsied each of the rats who lived on faulty diets, he found an incredible list of diseases—literally from head to tail.

The catalog of diseases he found in the animals included six types of lung disease, sinus trouble, ear trouble, adenoid growths, four different kinds of eye disease, eight varieties of gastrointestinal diseases, nine types of disease of the urinary tract including kidney stones, six different diseases of the male and female reproductive system, loss of hair, plus other skin problems, anemia, and other blood disorders, heart troubles galore, plus other diseases of the lymph glands, endocrine system, and nervous system. Whew!

Many of the diseases mentioned are not usually thought of as being due to poor nutrition. One of Dr. McCarrison's outstanding contributions to nutritional science was to prove that *poor nutrition sets the stage for the development of most diseases.*

NOTHING SO POTENT

"I know of nothing so potent in maintaining good health in laboratory animals as perfectly constituted food," concluded Dr. McCarrison. "I know of nothing so potent in producing ill health as improperly constituted food. This, too, is the experience of stockbreeders. Is man an exception to a rule so universally applicable to . . . animals?" [5]

Now, it would seem that an announcement by an important scientist that he had raised a group of disease-

5. Sir Robert McCarrison, *Nutrition and National Health*, p. 17. (London: Faber and Faber Limited, 1944.)

free rats would have made headlines throughout the world. You would think this would have become a major topic of conversation, and that further research would have been pushed to the ultimate to explore the consequences for you and for me. But things just don't seem to work that way.

Years ago, surgeons were so accustomed to pus and blood poisoning that they just took them for granted. When Dr. Joseph Lister first announced the results of antiseptic surgery, it caused very little stir among medical men. Many years were required before surgeons began to realize the importance of Lister's method of controlling infection. Have we similarly become too accustomed to disease and low standards of physical health?

Dr. McCarrison's laboratory at Coonoor was often visited by missionaries who were vacationing from the heat of the Nilgiri hills. He would tell them that he, too, was a missionary and that he had an appropriate text for his sermon. This was: "Harken diligently unto me, and eat ye that which is good" (Isaiah 55:2).

IS THIS YOUR DIET?

Dr. McCarrison also compared the diets of vigorous folks in northern India with the food used by many in the western world. He chose two groups of twenty rats each. One was fed a northern Indian diet, and the other had a diet he considered inadequate, overprocessed, and overcooked. The latter diet consisted of white bread, jam, margarine, tea with much sugar and little milk, boiled vegetables such as cabbage, potato, carrots, and so forth. In addition they got canned meat once a week.

"The first thing one noticed, as this experiment progressed," wrote Dr. McCarrison, "was that the members of the former, and well-fed, group lived happily together. They increased in weight and flourished. The other group did not increase in weight; their growth was stunted; they were badly proportioned; their coats were staring and lacking in gloss; they were nervous and apt to bite the attendants; they lived unhappily together and by the sixtieth day of the experiment they began to kill and eat the weaker ones amongst them. When they had disposed of three in this way, I was compelled to segregate the remainder." [6]

I suppose by now you are wondering what was in the healthful diet used by Dr. McCarrison. Since you probably buy your groceries in America, a description of their diet would be of little use to you. The approach to optimal nutrition described in this book *will show you how to get the benefits of the diet that brought such good results in Dr. McCarrison's experiment.*

FAULTY FOOD—FAULTY BODIES

Here is Dr. McCarrison's revolutionary conclusion: "The newer knowledge of nutrition has revealed, and reveals the more with every addition to it, that a chief cause of the physiological decay of organs and tissues of the body is faulty food, wherein deficiencies of some essentials are often combined with excesses of others. It is reasonable, then, to assume that dietetic malnutrition is a chief cause of many degenerative diseases of mankind." [7]

During the past week, you have probably been in contact with enough tuberculosis germs, pneumonia bacilli, and other assorted microbes and viruses to kill you. As you read this, billions of potentially deadly invaders are hammering away at your body. As long as

6. *Ibid.,* p. 24.
7. Sinclair, *op. cit.,* pp. 305-306.

your many defenses are working properly, these enemies are successfully fought off. When your resistance is low, bacteria or viruses will successfully gain a beachhead in your body. These invaders make their own replacements as they launch their attack. About every half-hour, they divide and you can be fighting twice as many. The possibilities are staggering—*a single germ could have a billion descendants in less than a day!* If your health is good, your body will wipe out every one of the invading enemies before they get a good start. Optimal nutrition has an indispensable part to play in helping you resist both degenerative and infectious diseases.

Medical education and practice, in general, have not kept abreast of the tremendous advances in nutritional knowledge, according to a survey by the Council of Foods and Nutrition of The American Medical Association.[8] Unfortunately, nutrition is all too often taught hurriedly as a rather simple thing in which, for example, a lack of vitamin A causes poor night vision, lack of B_1 causes beriberi, lack of vitamin C causes scurvy, lack of vitamin D causes rickets, etc. But remember the enormous number of diseases Dr. McCarrison found in his poorly fed rats. Most of these diseases are not associated with *the lack of single vitamins, minerals, proteins, fats, etc.* Dr. McCarrison's broad approach dealing *not with single nutrients but with nutrition as a whole over the lifetime as a whole* shows the vital connection between overall nutrition and overall health. Thanks to his efforts, we know today that the best way to fight disease is *not to fight disease, but to build the highest level of health through excellent nutrition.*

8. *Journal of the American Medical Association*, Vol. 183, p. 955, 1963.

Chapter 19

YOUR NUTRITION ANALYSIS

Your keen-minded participation in analyzing your diet is a vital part of this book. As you read this chapter, you will have an opportunity to find out how you have been treating your body. Your success in improving your nutrition will depend on how well we can work together on this. I am counting on you to do your part. Fair enough?

Now, let's start at the beginning. Years ago, at the moment of our conception, we were one-cell microscopic specks. Since that time, we've developed into complex human beings with about twenty-six trillion cells. Food made the difference. Every bit of our growth was produced by food and oxygen interacting with our hereditary makeup.

Approximately fifty known nutrients are needed by these twenty-six trillion cells in our bodies. If these nutrients are not present in our blood stream in proper amounts, we can suffer in one way or another. We may not sustain the highest possible energy level. Like McCarrison's rats, our bodies may develop diseases which we otherwise could have resisted if nutrition had been optimal. Also the period of our physical prime as indicated by fertility or virility may be reduced. Personality problems may arise as shown in the antisocial behavior of McCarrison's rats raised on an inadequate, overprocessed diet. Parts of our bodies may wear out sooner than necessary and our life span be shortened, as in the case of Dr. Sherman's rats on Diet A, receiving only an adequate diet instead of the improved Diet B.

YOUR NUTRITION ANALYSIS

"Health," said Franklin P. Adams, "is the thing that makes you feel that now is the best time of the year." Your first step in improving your health through nutrition is to evaluate your present diet. As an example of the Nutrition Analysis you will make for yourself, see Mr. V.I.P. Jr.'s analysis. He has listed all of the foods he used during the day and estimated the amount. The figures showing the percentage of the daily allowances for protein, vitamins, and minerals were taken from the Food Table which begins on page 217.

The figures in each column were then totaled so as to give him an overall picture of the nutritional value of his diet for the day. A total of 100 per cent exactly meets his recommended allowance for protein, vitamins, and minerals. Let's see how well he came out.

Notice that V.I.P. Jr.'s protein total came to 95 per cent of the National Research Council's daily allowance. His total of 28 per cent of life-stretching vitamin A was only about one-fourth the recommended allowance. He received 63 per cent of the allowance of vitamin B_1 and 60 per cent of the allowance for vitamin B_2. His intake of vitamin C was very low—only 14 per cent of the recommended allowance. He had a little over one-half the calcium they recommend, but his diet amply met the recommended allowance for iron.

NUTRITION ANALYSIS FORM

Name: _V. I. P., Jr._   Date: _____

FOOD	AMOUNT	PROTEIN	Vitamin A	Vitamin B₁	Vitamin B₂	Vitamin C	Calcium	Iron	Saturated Fat Calories	Total Fat Calories (Both saturated and unsaturated)	TOTAL CALORIES (From protein, fat, and carbohydrate)
Breakfast:											
Apple Juice	½ cup	0	1	2	2	1	1	6	0	0	62
Corn Flakes	1 oz.	3	0	8	2	0	0	5	0	2	110
Sugar	2 tbs.	0	0	0	0	0	0	0	0	0	100
White Bread	2 slices	6	0	8	6	0	4	12	8	18	120
Jelly	2 tbs.	0	0	0	0	2	0	2	0	0	100
Butter	2 pats	0	10	0	0	0	0	0	54	100	100
Coffee	1 cup	0	0	0	0	0	0	0	0	0	0
Mid-morning Snack:											
Cola Drink	8 oz.	0	0	0	0	0	0	0	0	0	105
Lunch:											
Hamburger with bun	1	21	0	10	7	0	6	27	44	97	254
Chocolate Cake	1 slice	7	3	2	6	0	15	5	45	126	420
Coffee	1 cup	0	0	0	0	0	0	0	0	0	0
Mid-afternoon:											
Ginger Ale	8 oz.	0	0	0	0	0	0	0	0	0	80
Sweet Chocolate Bar	2 oz.	2	0	2	4	0	4	16	54	144	270
Supper:											
Bean Soup	1 cup	11	0	6	6	0	12	28	18	45	190
Sirloin Steak	3 oz.	29	1	3	9	0	1	25	117	243	330
French Fried Potatoes	10 pieces	3	0	4	2	11	1	7	18	63	155
Rolls, soft	2	8	0	14	8	0	8	14	18	36	230
Butter	2 pats	0	10	0	0	0	0	0	54	100	100
Apple Brown Betty	½ cup	3	3	4	3	0	3	7	18	36	175
After Supper:											
Beer	1 can	2	0	0	5	0	2	0	0	3	171
DAILY TOTALS		95%	28%	63%	60%	14%	57%	154%	448	1,013	3,072

DIRECTIONS:
1. List on a separate line each food you ate in a typical day.
2. Estimate about how much you ate of each food. Write this amount in the second column.
3. Find each food in the Food Table and copy figures for the various nutrients into the proper columns.
4. If you ate half the amount shown in the Food Table, cut the various figures in half. If you ate double the quantity, then double each figure before writing it on this form, etc.
5. If you ate a prepared food not shown in the Food Table, list on a separate line each of the major ingredients in your portion of the recipe. Then look them up in the Food Table as you would for other foods.
6. If you used a food that is not shown in the Food Table, substitute figures for a food that is most like the one you ate.
7. Add all columns to get your daily intake of the various nutrients.

The significance of his 448 saturated fat calories and the 1,013 total fat calories were discussed in Chapter 7. Unfortunately, the amount of saturated fat and total fat in his diet are both high, and he may be heading for a coronary attack some day. Let's hope your Nutrition Analysis shows that your diet is better than his.

ANALYZING YOUR DIET

Someone once remarked that you can't do everything at once, but you can do *something* at once. Here, step by step, is the way to make a scientific analysis of your present diet to determine whether it is meeting the standards of the National Research Council:

1. Turn to one of the Nutrition Analysis Forms that follow the Food Table in the back of this book. List your typical day's diet in the column marked "Food." Each food you ate should be listed on a separate line.

2. Estimate the quantity that you used and write this amount in the proper column. This will become easier after you have done it a few times.

3. Look up each food in the Food Table beginning on page 217. Insert the figures for the various nutrients in the corresponding columns of your Nutrition Analysis Form.

4. IMPORTANT: If you ate one-half of the quantity that is shown in the Food Table, just cut all the figures in half. If you used double the amount shown in the Food Table, then double the figures. Page 211 contains additional information that may help you estimate quantities. After you have made several Nutrition Analyses, you will develop skill in estimating amounts of foods.

5. If a food you used is not listed, substitute the figures for a similar food. For example, if you ate a fruit that is not shown in the Food Table, substitute the figures for a fruit that is most like the one you ate.

6. If a prepared food was eaten that is not shown, list the ingredients in the recipe and look them up in the Food Table. List only the main ingredients of the recipe and do not include spices or condiments. Include in your Nutrition Analysis the figures for your portion of this recipe.

7. When you finish, add all columns to get an overall picture of your daily intake of the various nutrients.

In the next chapter you will find a Nutrition Test that will enable you to score yourself to find out how well you meet today's nutritional standards. *You cannot score yourself on this test until you complete your Nutrition Analysis Form as described above.*

EVALUATING YOUR TOTALS

Now let's see how well you are doing. The table on page 216 shows you the amount of protein, vitamins, and minerals recommended by the National Research Council. You will notice that they have slightly different allowances for men and women. The stresses of pregnancy and nursing require substantial increases in the women's allowances. This table also shows the daily totals that children and teenage boys and girls should have if their diet is to meet the recommendations of the National Research Council. When you compare your totals for protein, vitamins, and minerals with this table, you can determine whether you are meeting their standards of nutrition.

You will note that the National Research Council thus far has made no recommendations for the amount of saturated fat and total fat. Chapter 7 contains suggestions that can reduce your chances of a heart attack. You will recall that it was recommended that the total fat calories should not exceed 25 per cent of the total calories. The saturated fat in your diet should not exceed 6 per cent of your total calories.

The next page shows the Nutrition Analysis of a young doctor on a reducing diet. Notice how much nutrition he packed into only 1,703 calories! Note that his saturated fat was held to 6 per cent of his total calories and the total fat was about a fourth of the total calories.

YOU'RE ON YOUR WAY

As you analyze your diet, you will begin to think of foods in terms of the basic nutrients they offer you. You will see how your present diet stacks up against the recommendations of the National Research Council. By knowing your daily totals of protein, vitamins, minerals, fats, and calories, a new world of modern nutrition will open for you.

Although the cells of your body need about fifty nutrients continuously, it is, thank goodness, not necessary to check on all of these nutrients individually. For example, when you achieve the recommended allowance for protein, you will automatically take care of almost half of them. In general, a diet that contains adequate protein, plus vitamins A, B_1, B_2, C, calcium, iron, and fat will supply other nutrients in adequate amounts. This enormously simplifies our nutritional "bookkeeping."

Dr. George R. Minot of the Harvard Medical School has said, "Man's future will depend very largely upon what he decides to eat." Since much of your

NUTRITION ANALYSIS FORM

Name: _Young Doctor (Reducing Diet)_   Date: _____

FOOD	AMOUNT	PROTEIN	Vitamin A	Vitamin B_1	Vitamin B_2	Vitamin C	Calcium	Iron	Saturated Fat Calories	Total Fat Calories (Both saturated and unsaturated)	TOTAL CALORIES (From protein, fat, and carbohydrate)
Breakfast:											
Orange	1	1	6	8	2	88	8	3	0	2	70
Wheat Germ Cereal	1/2 cup	12	0	43	15	0	4	28	4	32	123
Bananas (sliced in cereal)	2	2	8	6	6	26	2	14	0	4	170
Beef Liver, fried	3 oz.	28	910	14	188	36	1	66	27	54	180
Skim Milk	2 cups	24	0	12	48	8	76	4	2	4	174
Mid-morning Snack:											
Peach	1	1	26	1	3	9	1	5	0	2	35
Lunch:											
Tomato Juice	1/2 cup	1	25	4	2	25	1	5	0	1	25
Cottage Cheese, creamed	1/2 cup	21	4	2	18	0	13	4	27	50	120
Tomato	1	3	33	5	3	47	2	9	0	2	30
Lettuce	1/4 head	2	12	3	5	12	3	6	0	2	17
Mayonnaise	1 tbs.	0	1	0	0	0	0	1	18	108	110
Buttermilk	1 cup	12	0	6	24	4	36	2	1	2	87
Mid-afternoon:											
Pear	1	1	1	2	4	9	2	5	1	9	100
Supper:											
Orange Juice, frozen	1/2 cup	1	5	7	1	75	1	1	0	1	55
Mackerel, broiled	3 oz.	27	9	8	13	0	1	10	23	117	200
Cole Slaw Salad	1/2 cup	1	1	2	1	33	3	2	4	32	50
Skim Milk	1 cup	12	0	6	24	4	38	2	1	2	87
Before Bed Snack:											
Apple	1	0	1	2	1	4	1	4	0	2	70
DAILY TOTALS		149%	1042%	151%	357%	358%	194%	171%	108	426	1,705

DIRECTIONS:

1. List on a separate line each food you ate in a typical day.
2. Estimate about how much you ate of each food. Write this amount in the second column.
3. Find each food in the Food Table and copy figures for the various nutrients into the proper columns.
4. If you ate half the amount shown in the Food Table, cut the various figures in half. If you ate double the quantity, then double each figure before writing it on this form, etc.
5. If you ate a prepared food not shown in the Food Table, list on a separate line each of the major ingredients in your portion of the recipe. Then look them up in the Food Table as you would for other foods.
6. If you used a food that is not shown in the Food Table, substitute figures for a food that is most like the one you ate.
7. Add all columns to get your daily intake of the various nutrients.

future may depend on what you decide to eat, it is important as a first step to find out *what you are now doing nutritionally*. You cannot score yourself on the interesting Nutrition Test in Chapter 20 until you know. It is most important that you list your typical daily diet and complete your Nutrition Analysis before you read further.

WHAT'S YOUR NUTRITION SCORE?

A friend once remarked to me as we were discussing optimal nutrition, "It must take a lot of will power."

"No," I pointed out, "it's not a matter of will power. It's more a matter of understanding. When you become fascinated with achieving the highest possible level of buoyant energy, the least amount of sickness, and a vigorous long life, you probably won't need will power to force yourself."

Health is the first wealth. When you experience the difference that modern nutrition can make, you acquire an eagerness and deep satisfaction in improving your diet toward optimal levels. This can be enjoyable and esthetically pleasing—but you must be smart enough to first blast yourself out of a nutritional rut and learn to use the more nutritious foods in ways that are acceptable to you.

As you have probably noticed, many foods offer you only a modest contribution toward your daily percentage of the various nutrients. But every now and then you'll run into a food in which a single serving provides you with about a day's supply of a nutrient. For example, notice that a small glass of fresh orange juice will provide 81 per cent of your daily allowance for vitamin C. One-half cup of turnip greens, if not overcooked, will supply 154 per cent of your vitamin A plus 58 per cent of your allowance for vitamin C.

It will pay you to study the Food Table thoroughly. Mark boldly any foods that supply unusual amounts of two or more nutrients. Three ounces of a certain food not only supplies 28 per cent of the protein allowance, but also provides 910 per cent of the vitamin A, 14 per cent of the vitamin B_1, 188 per cent of the vitamin B_2, 36 per cent of the vitamin C, and 66 per cent of the iron! Have you noticed this wonderful food and the many other foods that supply large amounts of several nutrients?

Dorothy M. Youland tells us, "Nutrition is the most important single factor affecting health. This is true at age 1 or 101." [1] Progress in your adventure toward optimal nutrition will depend to a large extent on how rapidly you discover what foods are the most nutritious. You will then be able to gradually modify your diet *in a balanced way* to include the more nutritious foods and exclude "empty" foods that contain mainly calories, but offer very little of the other vital nutrients. Consider this a workbook, and don't hesitate to mark it up in ways that make it more useful to you. A well-marked book may be a lifetime companion.

WHAT'S YOUR NUTRITION SCORE?

At the end of this chapter you will find an interesting Nutrition Test that will enable you to check up on yourself. Your score on this test will tell you how well you meet today's accepted nutritional standards. V.I.P. Jr.'s diet shown on page 185 scored rather poorly on this test. He scored only 58 points out of a

1. Dorothy M. Youland, "New Dimensions for Public Health Nutrition," *American Journal of Clinical Nutrition*, Vol. 9, p. 211, 1961.

possible 100. That's awful! Let's hope you beat him.

The Nutrition Test is based on the recommendations of the top authorities in the United States. The items for scoring your protein, vitamin, and mineral intakes are based on the recommended allowances of the National Research Council. Your score on items eight and nine will enable you to tell whether you are getting too much saturated fat and too much total fat in your diet, which might someday lead to trouble. This part of the Test uses the recommendations of Dr. Ancel Keys of the University of Minnesota. He has intensively studied the relationship between too much fat and coronary heart attacks.

The last item in the test will enable you to determine whether you are carrying around too many excess pounds. As discussed in Chapter 2, the longer your waistline, the shorter your lifeline. This part of the test is based on the latest "Desirable Weight Tables" of the Metropolitan Life Insurance Company.

To find your Nutrition Score on the test that follows, it will be necessary for you to have completed your Nutrition Analysis as described in the last chapter. If you had any difficulty making this analysis for yourself, it may help to study the Nutrition Analysis of V.I.P. Jr. that appears on page 185 and read the previous chapter again. A second reading will help you pick up points that could easily have been missed on the first go-round.

At this point you should be ready to take the Nutrition Test. If you score 100 points, you are meeting today's accepted standards of nutrition—congratulations! Most people score only around 60 to 70 points. They have a long way to go to meet today's accepted nutritional standards—to say nothing of the optimal levels that we will discuss later in this book.

You are now ready to take the Nutrition Test. Good luck to you!

WHAT'S YOUR NUTRITION SCORE?

1. Protein Intake: From the totals of your Daily Nutrition Analysis find your daily percentage of the protein allowance and score yourself as follows:

Men		Women		
100% or above	25 points	83% or above	25 points	
90% to 99%	20 points	75% to 82%	20 points	
80% to 89%	15 points	66% to 74%	15 points	
70% to 79%	10 points	58% to 65%	10 points	
60% to 69%	5 points	50% to 57%	5 points	
Below 60%	0 points	Below 50%	0 points	Protein Score_____

2. Vitamin A: Find your daily percentage of vitamin A and score yourself as shown in the table below:

Men and Women

100% or above	5 points	70% to 79%	2 points	
90% to 99%	4 points	60% to 69%	1 point	
80% to 89%	3 points	Below 60%	0 points	Vitamin A Score_____

3. Vitamin B_1: Find your daily percentage of vitamin B_1 and score yourself as shown in the table below:

Men		Women		
100% or above	5 points	75% or above	5 points	
90% to 99%	4 points	68% to 74%	4 points	
80% to 89%	3 points	60% to 67%	3 points	
70% to 79%	2 points	53% to 59%	2 points	
60% to 69%	1 point	45% to 52%	1 point	
Below 60%	0 points	Below 45%	0 points	Vitamin B_1 Score_____

4. Vitamin B_2 Find your daily percentage of vitamin B_2 and score yourself as shown in the table below:

Men		Women		
100% or above	5 points	83% or above	5 points	
90% to 99%	4 points	75% to 82%	4 points	
80% to 89%	3 points	66% to 74%	3 points	
70% to 79%	2 points	58% to 65%	2 points	
60% to 69%	1 point	50% to 57%	1 point	
Below 60%	0 points	Below 50%	0 points	Vitamin B_2 Score_____

5. Vitamin C: Find your daily percentage of vitamin C and score yourself as shown in the table below:

Men		Women		
100% or above	5 points	93% or above	5 points	
90% to 99%	4 points	84% to 92%	4 points	
80% to 89%	3 points	75% to 83%	3 points	
70% to 79%	2 points	65% to 74%	2 points	
60% to 69%	1 point	56% to 64%	1 point	
Below 60%	0 points	Below 56%	0 points	Vitamin C Score_____

6. Calcium: Find your daily percentage of calcium and score yourself as shown in the table below:

Men and Women

100% or above	5 points	70% to 79%	2 points	
90% to 99%	4 points	60% to 69%	1 point	
80% to 89%	3 points	Below 60%	0 points	Calcium Score_____

7. Iron: Score your daily iron percentage as follows:

Men		Women	
100% or above	5 points	120% or above	5 points
90% to 99%	4 points	108% to 119%	4 points
80% to 89%	3 points	96% to 107%	3 points
70% to 79%	2 points	84% to 95%	2 points
60% to 69%	1 point	72% to 83%	1 point
Below 60%	0 points	Below 72%	0 points

Iron Score _____

8. Amount of Saturated Fat Calories: Find your saturated fat calories in your Nutrition Analysis Form. Score as follows:

Men		Women	
200 or less	10 points	145 or less	10 points
201 to 270	8 points	146 to 195	8 points
271 to 340	6 points	196 to 245	6 points
341 to 410	4 points	246 to 295	4 points
411 to 480	2 points	296 to 345	2 points
Over 480	0 points	Over 345	0 points

Saturated Fat Score_____

9. Amount of Total Fat Calories: Find your total fat calories in your Nutrition Analysis Form. Score as follows:

Men		Women	
800 or less	10 points	575 or less	10 points
801 to 900	8 points	576 to 647	8 points
901 to 1000	6 points	648 to 720	6 points
1001 to 1100	4 points	721 to 792	4 points
1101 to 1200	2 points	793 to 865	2 points
Over 1200	0 points	Over 865	0 points

Total Fat Score_____

10. Desirable Weight: Find the desirable weight range for your height and body build in the Desirable Weight Table on page 10. If you are within your indicated weight range, score 25 points. For every pound above your desirable weight range, subtract 1 point from the 25 points you can score on this item. If you are 25 pounds or more over your weight range, score 0.

Weight Score _____

Add All Your Scores Together.
A perfect score on this test is 100.

Total Nutrition Score_____

Chapter 21

THE CHALLENGE OF OPTIMAL NUTRITION

In 1927, 710 people who lived in a slum area were moved into a new municipal housing project. The housing authorities wanted to show that the improved sanitation and greater amount of room in the new project would result in a higher level of health. The health records of these 710 people had been kept during the previous five years, when they lived in crowded slums. A continuing record of their health was maintained for the first five years after they moved into the fine new project. Health records of another group of people who continued to live in a slum area were kept for comparison.

The authorities were astounded to find that people who moved into the new housing project had a higher death rate! The yearly rate increased from 23 deaths per 1,000 people in the slums to about 34 deaths per 1,000 in the new housing project. This was almost a 50 per cent higher death rate! The death rate of those who remained in the slum area did not increase during this period.[1]

1. G. C. M. McGonigle and J. Kirby, *Poverty and Public Health.* (London: Victor Gollanez, Ltd., 1937.)

This shocking result led to further investigation. Why were people healthier living in crowded slums? They found that when these folks moved from the slums, their rental was almost doubled. The pinch on their budget gave them less money to spend on food. This higher death rate might not have occurred if these people had known what you know about working toward optimal nutrition.

Food is one of the largest items in the budget of most families. Some people I've talked with have wondered if they would be able to afford a program of optimal nutrition. Actually they cannot afford to be without it. Doctor's and dentist's bills, hospital expenses, and the time lost from work may ruin your budget. Most people are pleasantly surprised to learn that an optimal diet is not necessarily an expensive diet.

NUTRITION AND ECONOMY

The Food Table is the key to planning nutritious meals that will fit into your budget. This table gives you scientific information on the health-building values of foods—free from advertising hocus-pocus.

Protein is usually considered one of the most expensive of the nutrients. It can be quite inexpensive, provided you do not insist on getting it from sirloin steak. For example, the recommended daily allowance of protein obtained from sirloin steak at a dollar a pound costs about ninety-four cents. A day's supply of protein from nonfat skim milk powder at nine cents per quart costs about eighteen cents. Thus the top-quality protein in skim milk powder costs far less. But note that skim milk powder contains four times more B_1, six times more B_2, and eighty-eight times more calcium! And the nonfat milk has practically none of the potentially dangerous saturated fat with which sirloin steak is loaded. This is only one example of how an intelligent nutrition-conscious person, armed with the Food Table, can get more nutritional value from each dollar spent for food.

It is interesting to note that usually the more nutritious the food, the lower its cost! Liver, kidneys, and other organ meats of animals are less expensive than muscle meats, and yet they are far higher in vitamins and minerals and lower in saturated fats. Wheat germ, which is the most nutritious cereal, is a real bargain. Five cents worth of wheat germ (priced at two and three-quarter cents an ounce) furnishes 18 per cent of the daily recommended allowance for protein. When compared with a nickel's worth of corn flakes (at two cents an ounce), wheat germ offers two and one-half times more protein (and it's complete protein, too), three times more vitamin B_1, over five times more vitamin B_2, and three times more iron. In addition it contains wheat germ oil—a valuable unsaturated fat and the richest source of vitamin E. [2]

Other protein bargains are cottage cheese, domestic sardines, and soybeans. Soybeans may be made into a tasty soybean loaf, soybean croquettes, sandwich spreads, etc. The excellent book by Dr. Philip Chen, entitled *Soybeans for Health, Longevity, and Economy,* has many interesting recipes for using this valuable food.

Dr. Clive McCay of Cornell University has said, "Our daily paper would surprise us if it carried an ad: 'Wanted: a vegetable that will grow in any climate, rivals meat in nutritive value, matures in three or five days, may be planted any day in the year, requires neither soil nor sunshine, rivals tomatoes in vitamin C, has no waste, can be cooked with as little fuel and as quickly as a pork chop.' " The Chinese discovered this

2. Printed in 1966! Prices are higher today but these foods are still proportionately more economical.

vegetable many centuries ago—bean sprouts grown from mung beans.

On a small tray in my kitchen I have six plastic containers that produce a quart of bean sprouts each day. These sprouts with cottage cheese make a delicious salad. They can be steamed with onions and served as a gourmet hot dish with soy sauce. You can grow a year-round supply of fresh nutritious mung bean sprouts at a cost of only five cents per quart. When I eat these crunchy sprouts I have the satisfaction of knowing they are living-fresh when they go into my mouth. I don't have to allow for possible loss of vitamin C due to wilting. It is also nice to know that they contain no insecticide residues whose long-term effects, according to Dr. James McLester and Dr. William Darby, "may be a potential source of danger." [3] Since these delicious vegetables are grown in my kitchen rather than under open skies, they probably have a minimum of radioactive strontium 90.

You'll be delighted by the way your knowledge of nutrition will help you get more for your food dollar. By using the Food Table as a guide to nutritive values, you are now equipped to make intelligent comparisons among the myriad of foods facing you on the market shelves. You'll probably find that you can enjoy the benefits of improved nutrition *on less than you are now spending!*

HOW DISEASES MAY START

"There is probably no other single factor so important to the achievement and maintenance of health

3. James S. McLester and William J. Darby, *Nutrition and Diet in Health and Disease*, 6th ed., p. 352. (Philadelphia: W. B. Saunders Company, 1952.)

as nutrition," says Dr. Robert E. Shank of the Washington University School of Medicine. Let us consider how faulty nutrition can bring about the large number of diseases that do so much to wreck our budgets and shatter our happiness. Dr. Norman Jolliffe in his classic work, *Clinical Nutrition,* has pointed out that there are two sources of poor nutrition:

1. We may fail to eat the things we should. This could be due to inadequate knowledge of nutrition, to food allergies, the nausea of pregnancy, or other factors.

2. We may fail to absorb properly the food we eat. This could be due to inadequate digestive secretions, diarrhea, use of mineral oil, or other factors.

When our nutrition is inadequate for either of the above reasons, our nutrient reserves will be used up. We can, for example, store a year's supply of vitamin A, but only a few day's supply of vitamins B_1, B_2, or C. When these reserves are gone, we will soon be depleted of the nutrients needed continuously by our cells and tissues. This leads to *biochemical lesions.* This means that the complex chemical reactions inside our bodies that keep us going cannot take place in the best possible way. Biochemical lesions may gradually make *functional changes* which, according to Dr. Jolliffe, "include such common complaints as excessive fatigability, disturbances in sleep, inability to concentrate, 'gas,' heart consciousness, and various queer bodily sensations." [4]

If poor nutrition continues after functional changes take place, your body structure may begin to deteriorate in various ways. These could include dry and crinkled skin, cracks at the corners of the lips, bleeding gums, a tendency to bruise easily, changes in the tongue, the white part of the eyes becomes infiltrated with blood

4. Norman Jolliffe, "The Pathogenesis of Deficiency Disease," from Norman Jolliffe, F. F. Tisdall, and Paul R. Cannon, eds., *Clinical Nutrition,* p. 33; see also pp. 3-38. (New York: Hoeber Medical Division, Harper & Row, Publishers, Inc., 1950.)

vessels and gives a bloodshot appearance, granulated eyelids, etc. *Insidious deterioration will also take place in vital internal organs where it cannot be seen.*

Poor nutrition is usually discovered only when you look like you're headed downhill. But as we can see from Dr. Jolliffe's analysis, such obvious changes are *only the last stage in a downward spiral of interacting events leading to deteriorating health.* Frequently a program that approaches optimal nutrition can reverse these changes—but sometimes too much damage has occurred to be repaired.

The goal of this book has been to show you how to nourish your body so well that you should never start on that tragic downward spiral in which:

1. Your nutrition is inadequate so that
2. your nutrient reserves are used up and
3. your tissues are depleted leading to
4. biochemical lesions which bring on
5. functional changes which can in turn result in
6. physical deterioration.

By following the path toward optimal nutrition, you should be able to meet the golden years of your life with vigor and health. Your body should be able to make the most of its inborn potentialities for a long, worthwhile life.

WE CONTINUOUSLY CHANGE

For years it had been assumed that once we were grown, about all we had to do was to supply our bodies with enough calories for fuel and enough of the other nutrients for repairs when we bang up a knee or get our fingers caught in a door. The use of radioactive tracers has shown that such a static picture of our bodies is completely wrong. An adult body changes every second. If you wish to understand the great significance of optimal nutrition for you, you must learn to view your body as a *rapidly changing dynamic organism.*

"Life," said the sage, "is a grindstone. Whether it polishes you up or grinds you down depends on you." Similarly, the millions of small changes that take place every second in your body may help to build your health to higher levels, or may represent a gradual but cumulative deterioration. Whether you are going up or down can depend on whether you provide optimal amounts of the fifty nutrients that are needed daily by the twenty-six trillion hungry cells of your body.

Research with radioactive "tagged" atoms has shown that even your bones are not the permanent solid things they were once thought to be. Calcium, phosphorus, magnesium, and other minerals continuously dissolve from your bones and whether they are properly replaced depends on your nutrition. About every twenty days, there is a turnover of about one per cent of the calcium in the bones in your body!

How rapidly is the *protein* in our bodies changing? By using radioactive tracers, scientists have shown that the protein in your body is constantly being broken down and replaced. There is a continuous interchange between the amino acids in your tissues and the circulating amino acids in your blood.[5] It has been estimated that about every eighty days one-half of your body protein is replaced![6] This turnover is most rapid in your liver and blood, and these two account for about 41 per cent of the total exchange.

This means that when you work toward an optimal diet, you provide your body with a generous supply of first-rate materials needed to rebuild in the finest possible way. Since about one per cent of the protein in

5. R. Schoenheimer, *The Dynamic State of Body Constituents.* (Cambridge: Harvard University, 1942.)

6. D. B. Sprinson and D. Rittenberg, *Journal of Biological Chemistry*, Vol. 180, p. 715, 1949.

your body is turned over every three days, and about one per cent of the calcium in your bones is turned over every twenty days, you can see that your body may, in a small but cumulative way, begin to benefit immediately through improved nutrition.

Do not, however, be impatient. Years of going downhill cannot be corrected quickly through a few mouthfuls of wholesome 'food. It has been my experience that most people will notice some benefits from a program of optimal nutrition within one month. Many of the added health benefits come only after four to six months or longer.

FOR A LONG LIFE

Dr. Clive McCay of Cornell has extensively studied relationships between aging and nutrition. From his experiments which spanned several decades, he has made the following practical suggestions for those who seek the highest level of health:

> Mechanization has decreased human movement so that the typical older person can live with very little compulsory exercise. Hence his intake of foods in terms of energy usually will amount to only 1,500 to 2,000 calories or about half the intake of an adult or a large youth. With this lowered intake of food every effort must be made to insure high quality in terms of essentials, because the need for such elements as calcium does not decline in proportion to the need for energy. In fact the requirement for calcium rises in old age and may exceed the amount needed at any other period of life. Likewise the need for vitamins and protein seems just as high in old age as in middle life.
>
> The second great hazard in later life is the

temptation to consume foods that provide little beside energy. The two that create the greatest danger are alcohol and sugar. The next two in order of importance are cooking fats and white flour. With the exception of alcohol these substances all offer the additional temptation of being cheap sources of energy. They are not cheap if they lead to years of ill health in later life. . . .

Since the old person may be dependent upon foods ready to eat he should give special attention to basic products such as bread. Bread can be made from excellent formulas containing milk, wheat germ, soy flour and yeast, or it can be made very poorly of white flour with few additions. What is true for bread is also true for breakfast cereals and sweet baked goods.

The older person can help his own diet by mixing dry skim milk or dry yeast into his foods. He can keep a sugar bowl on his table filled with powdered bone meal and another filled with yeast or wheat germ. These supplements can be eaten at each meal. Milk is probably the best food for later life. Tests with animals have indicated that they can be reared and kept for the whole of life upon no other food than fresh milk. Older as well as younger people can profit by the use of more milk. . . .

Nutrition during later life requires regular study by every individual to insure sound food habits and avoid the pitfalls of alcohol, sugar and fat.[7]

7. Clive M. McCay, "Chemical Aspects of Ageing and the Effect of Diet Upon Ageing," from Albert I. Lansing, ed., *Problems of Ageing*, 3rd ed., pp. 192-193. (Baltimore: The Williams and Wilkins Company, 1952.)

KEEP UP TO DATE

Thomas Jefferson once expressed the hope that newspapers might someday classify their news under the headings *facts, probabilities, possibilities,* and *lies.* I have tried to make this book rich in facts, for these are the bricks out of which theories are built. All scientific theories should be regarded as probabilities—not certainties. Cassius J. Keyser said, "Absolute certainty is the privilege of uneducated minds—and fanatics. It is, for scientific folks, an unattainable ideal."

I have tried to make it clear throughout this book that our suggestions for optimal human nutrition must at this time be classified under "probabilities" and "possibilities." Although this book contains no deliberate lies, nutrition today is such a young science that future research will almost certainly result in revisions of some parts of present nutritional information. It will pay you to keep your antenna up and to subscribe to one or more magazines that will put you in touch with current nutritional findings. A list of suggested further readings is given on pages 208 to 210.

THE PROMISE OF OPTIMAL NUTRITION

Dr. Sherman has often remarked on the tragedy of a short "prime of life." By the time we get the mortgage on our home paid off and develop a degree of wisdom and maturity, our lives may be about over. When the experience of a great industrial leader or a great statesman has accumulated to the point where he is able to make important contributions to society, he often has tragically little time left. Dr. Sherman was elated when his experiments with rats on Diet B showed that the prime of life could be lengthened by improved nutrition.

"There is no cure for birth or death, save to enjoy the interval," said philosopher George Santayana. Optimal nutrition is needed to participate in life to its fullest. The added energy and health you may receive can enable you to do things that you would never have tackled otherwise. After a hard day's work, it may help you fill your evening with deeply satisfying and productive experiences. Instead of collapsing into an easy chair near the TV set, you may be at your best for new achievements. People will notice the added spring to your step, and a greater feeling of vitality will be evident in most things that you do. Sometimes improved nutrition not only enables people to feel and act younger, but it also makes them look younger.

Your program of optimal nutrition can be one of the most exciting adventures of your life. It can be as fascinating as any deep-sea treasure hunt. It can be as interesting as any business deal pulled off by great industrial leaders. Helping your body overcome health problems that have been nagging you for years can be as thrilling as any detective mystery. In doing your part to help America build strong and healthy future generations, you will be meeting your highest and most solemn obligation of citizenship. To help others build up their bodies and thus live happier lives can be as soul-satisfying as any great deed. This challenge and opportunity are now yours, for as Dr. Henry Sherman said, "Nutrition is everyone's adventure."

Your knowledge of nutrition is now up to date. And now it's up to you!

APPENDICES

Appendix *I*

FOR FURTHER STUDY

A number of excellent cookbooks written by nutrition-conscious authors are now available. Their recipes are designed to preserve vitamins and minerals, increase the amount of protein, hold down on saturated fat and total fat, substitute liquid fats for solid fats, and to emphasize the choice of the more nutritious ingredients.

The following is a list of books that may provide you with signposts on your road to optimal nutrition:

Common Herbs for Natural Health, Juliette de Bairacli Levy (New York: Schocken Books, 1974). This book can introduce you to the fascinating field of how to use natural herbs in place of drugstore medicine for various health problems. It suggests many herbs that may be helpful in assisting your body to do its inner work to keep you healthy.

Eat Well and Stay Well, Ancel and Margaret Keys (New York: Doubleday & Co., Inc., 1963). This book contains a discussion of fat and coronary heart trouble by one of the world's top authorities. Dr. Keys' wife, Margaret, has included over 200 recipes that have been especially designed to assist you in working toward an optimal amount of fat in your diet.

Food Pollution, the Violation of Our Inner Ecology, Gene Marine and Judith Van Allen (New York: Holt, Rinehart and Winston, 1972). This book documents how our foods are commercially processed with various chemicals designed to make them taste better, have a longer shelf life, look better and cost less, with little or no understanding of the possible long-term effects on our health and longevity. Since food additives must now appear on labels, this book can tell you what to look for.

Journal of the American Dietetic Association (Published monthly by the American Dietetic Association, 620 North Michigan Avenue, Chicago, Illinois, $18 per year subscription price). This journal is written for those in the profession, but you may be able to benefit by some of the articles if you have *thoroughly absorbed* the nutritional information in this book. One of the features is a review of current literature that abstracts the latest nutritional findings from medical and scientific journals throughout the world.

Low-Fat Cookery, Evelyn S. Stead and Gloria K. Warren (Arc Books, 1972). This book contains many recipes designed to help you prepare delicious foods with a minimum of fat.

The Natural Foods Cookbook, Beatrice Trum Hunter (Pyramid Publications, 1972). This book contains nearly 1,200 recipes which emphasize the preparation and use of unusually nutritious foods. The introduction was written by Dr. Clive M. McCay of Cornell University and his wife, Jeannette B. McCay, both of whom specialize in nutrition.

Soybeans for Health and a Longer Life, Philip S. Chen (Keats, 1973). This book has many recipes for using the low cost, high quality protein of soybeans in breads, cakes, cookies, pies, soups, entrees, etc.

The kitchen of the Cornucopia Institute has a book shelf containing a number of cookbooks. The kitchen staff advises me that the following books are used most frequently:

Diet for a Small Planet, Frances Moore Lappe (New York: A Friends of the Earth/Ballantine Book, 1971). This book contains a lot of information on how to get protein from vegetable sources, with special emphasis on combining foods to create complete protein.

Let's Cook It Right, Adelle Davis (New York: Harcourt Brace Jovanovich, Inc., 1970). This excellent cookbook is a gold mine of information on preparing highly nutritious meals.

Tassajara Bread Book, Edward Espe Brown (Berkeley: Shambala Publications, Inc., 1973). This wonderful book tells how to bake our own nutritious bread, pastry, pancakes, muffins, cookies, and even candies.

Tassajara Cooking, Edward Espe Brown (Berkeley: Shambala Publications, Inc., 1973). This delightfully illustrated book shares the nutritious vegetarian recipes used at Tassajara, a Zen Mountain Center near Big Sur, California.

Ten Talents, Frank J. Hurd and Rosalie Hurd (Chisholm, Minn.: Dr. and Mrs. Frank J. Hurd, 1968). This beautifully prepared cookbook helps you combine good nutrition with enjoyment in cooking and eating.

Cosmic Cookery, Kathryn Hannaford (Berkeley: Starmast Publications, 1974). A great cookbook that will show you how good tasting you can make really nutritious food.

The Farm Vegetarian Cookbook, (Summertown, Tenn.: The Book Publishing Company, 1975). This cookbook contains favorites used on *The Farm* in Tennessee. Be sure to try their tofu-spinach pie.

The New York Times Natural Foods Cookbook, Jean Hewitt (New York: Avon Books, 1971). A standard reference cookbook that contains recipes for almost everything.

USING THE FOOD TABLE

After you've used the Food Table a few times, you will develop an ability to estimate food quantities. It will help you get started if you take a measuring cup from the kitchen and try checking out a half-cup, three-quarters cup, and a whole cup of various foods you eat. Whenever measures are given, such as a tablespoon or a cup, it should be understood that these refer to *level* tablespoons and *level* cups. The following information may be helpful to you in converting the values in the Food Table to the quantities that you use:

$$1 \text{ quart} = 32 \text{ fluid ounces}$$
$$= 4 \text{ cups}$$
$$1 \text{ pint} = 16 \text{ fluid ounces}$$
$$= 2 \text{ cups}$$
$$1 \text{ cup} = 8 \text{ fluid ounces}$$
$$= \frac{1}{2} \text{ pint}$$
$$= 16 \text{ tablespoons}$$
$$2 \text{ tablespoons} = 1 \text{ fluid ounce}$$
$$3 \text{ teaspoons} = 1 \text{ tablespoon}$$
$$16 \text{ ounces} = 1 \text{ pound}$$

It is not essential that you be meticulously precise to do a good job of analyzing your daily nutritional intake. Nutritionists who calculate the value of a day's meal and compare their values with the results of chemical analysis, often find that there is an error of about 10 per cent when food tables are used. This is because foods may vary from the average values given in the Food Table. Some varieties of fruits and vegetables are higher than shown in the Food Table. Others may be lower.

For those who wish to be more exact, you'll find the weight of each food in tenths of an ounce in the Table, except for those given in fluid ounces. If there are any doubts about quantities, you can always weigh foods to make sure that the quantity you are using is comparable to that in the Food Table. The weights shown apply to the whole food, but the nutrient figures apply only to the parts customarily eaten. For example, the weight figures for watermelon include rind and seeds—but the nutrient figures only refer to the part generally eaten.

DEVELOP THE ABILITY TO MAKE REASONABLE SUBSTITUTIONS

Don't get stumped if a food you use does not appear in this Food Table. No table that has ever been prepared covers all foods or all forms of any food. If the table shows figures for a fresh fruit and you used canned fruit, use the fresh values. The differences will not be great. If you ate a vegetable that is not listed in the Food Table, figure out what vegetable is most like it and use its values. You may be a little high in one column and a bit low in another, but the long-run percentage of error will probably cancel out to an insignificant amount. If a table were sufficiently complete to cover every food you are likely to eat in every way it is usually prepared, it could easily contain 10,000 items and thus be hopelessly complicated. Our Food Table contains over 750 entries and that's enough.

TECHNICAL INFORMATION

Some readers who have studied nutrition may be interested in knowing something of the scientific background of our Table. Most of the data in this Food Table has been taken from the *Home and Garden Bulletin No.* 72 of the United States Department of Agriculture. Some figures came from *Composition of Foods —Raw, Processed, Prepared*, also published by the Department. Several of the figures are from university research departments or industry sources. A few items shown as "cooked" were calculated from raw weights with an allowance for destruction of vitamin B_1, vitamin C, and changes in weight.

The percentages of protein, vitamins, and minerals have been based upon the recommended daily allowances of the National Research Council (1958 revision) for a 154-pound 25-year-old American man who is moderately active. Any daily diet that adds up to 100 per cent in protein, vitamins, and minerals will theoretically contain the following amounts of the various nutrients:

Nutrient	*Amount*
Protein	70 grams
Vitamin A	5,000 international units
Vitamin B_1 (thiamine)	1.6 milligrams
Vitamin B_2 (riboflavin)	1.8 milligrams
Vitamin C (ascorbic acid)	75 milligrams
Calcium	800 milligrams
Iron	10 milligrams

In 1964 the National Research Council revised their recommended daily allowances. They reduced the allowance on vitamin B_1, B_2, and vitamin C—the three water-soluble vitamins. The allowance on B_1 was lowered 25 per cent, B_2 about 6 per cent and vitamin C about 7 per cent. These water-soluble vitamins are constantly being removed from the blood stream by the filtering action of the kidneys. They are readily lost when vegetables and fruits are soaked or boiled. Of the three, vitamin C is particularly perishable. The author does not feel that our quest for optimal nutrition will be aided by reducing our intake of water-soluble vitamins as shown in the 1964 revision of the National Research Council's recommended daily allowances. This is why the Food Table is based on the 1958 allowances instead of the 1964 allowances.

THE VITAMIN-MINERAL INDEX

The Vitamin-Mineral Index is designed to show the average contribution in vitamins and minerals that each food makes to your diet. The Index is not dependent on the quantity of food eaten. Gasoline may be rated at hundred-octane whether you use one gallon or a hundred. In like manner, the Vitamin-Mineral Index of a food is a constant figure that can be validly compared with the Index of other foods. When a food has a Vitamin-Mineral Index twice as high as another food, it gives you *on the average* twice as many vitamins and minerals.

For those with a scientific frame of mind, here's how you can compute the Vitamin-Mineral Index of any food.

1. Find the amount of vitamins A, B_1, B_2, C, and the minerals calcium and iron in a given quantity of the food.

2. Using the recommended daily allowances of the National Research Council for a 154-pound moderately active man, compute the percentages of the allowance for each of the above nutrients supplied by the quantity of food chosen.

3. Add up these six percentages and divide by six to get the average percentage supplied by this quantity of the food.

4. Divide the calories in the quantity of food chosen into the average percentage and multiply that result by one hundred. This is the Vitamin-Mineral Index of that particular food.

5. The Vitamin-Mineral Index computed according to the above instructions will give you the average percentage of the National Research Council's recommended daily allowance for the above six nutrients supplied by a hundred-calorie portion.

Appendix *III*

RECOMMENDED ALLOWANCES FOR VARIOUS GROUPS

If the daily totals on your Nutrition Analysis Form add up to the percentages shown for your group, your diet meets the recommended allowances of the National Research Council.

Group	Protein	Vit. A	Vit. B$_1$	Vit. B$_2$	Vit. C	Calcium	Iron
Man, 25 years old, weighing 154 pounds	100%	100%	100%	100%	100%	100%	100%
Woman, 25 years old, weighing 128 pounds	83%	100%	75%	83%	93%	100%	120%
*Pregnant woman (2nd half)	111%	120%	81%	111%	133%	188%	150%
*Nursing woman	140%	160%	106%	139%	200%	250%	150%
*Children:							
1- 3 years (27 lbs.)	57%	40%	44%	56%	47%	125%	70%
4- 6 years (40 lbs.)	71%	50%	56%	72%	67%	125%	80%
7- 9 years (60 lbs.)	86%	70%	69%	83%	80%	125%	100%
10-12 years (79 lbs.)	100%	90%	81%	100%	100%	150%	120%
*Boys:							
13-15 years (108 lbs.)	121%	100%	100%	117%	120%	175%	150%
16-19 years (139 lbs.)	143%	100%	113%	139%	133%	175%	150%
*Girls:							
13-15 years (108 lbs.)	114%	100%	81%	111%	107%	163%	150%
16-19 years (120 lbs.)	107%	100%	75%	106%	107%	163%	150%

*400 units daily of vitamin D are recommended.

(Based on the values of the Food Table and Recommended Dietary Allowances, Revised 1958, National Research Council.)

216

Appendix IV

HEALTH-BUILDING VALUES OF FOODS

FOOD	AMOUNT	PROTEIN	Vitamin A	Vitamin B_1	Vitamin B_2	Vitamin C	Calcium	Iron	Saturated Fat Calories	Total Fat Calories (Both saturated and unsaturated)	TOTAL CALORIES (From protein, fat, and carbohydrate)	V-M INDEX	REMARKS (The Vitamin-Mineral Index is shown at left. The higher the Index number, the more vitamins and minerals per calorie of food.)
Acerola fruit, pitted	3.5 oz.	1	0	1	3	2419	1	2	0	3	30	1349	Tops in vitamin C.
Acerola juice	1/2 cup (4 fl. oz.)	1	1	2	3	2356	1	5	0	0	27	1462	By far the richest source of vitamin C.
Ale	1 can (12 fl. oz.)	2	0	2	6	0	6	3	0	0	148	2	
Almonds, shelled	14 almonds (1/2 oz.)	4	0	2	7	0	4	7	5	69	85	4	Has complete protein and desirable unsaturated fat.
Angel food cake	2" sector of 8" diam. cake (1.4 oz.)	4	0	0	3	0	1	1	0	2	110	1	
Apple	1 medium, 2-1/2" diam. (5.3 oz.)	0	1	2	1	4	1	4	0	2	70	3	Excellent in place of high calorie desserts.
Apple juice	1/2 cup (4 fl. oz.)	0	0	2	2	1	1	6	0	0	62	3	
Applesauce: Unsweetened	1/2 cup (4.2 oz.)	0	1	2	1	2	1	5	0	1	50	4	
Sweetened	1/2 cup (4.5 oz.)	0	1	1	1	2	1	5	0	1	92	2	Sweetening almost doubles the calories.
Apple brown betty	1/2 cup (4.1 oz.)	3	3	4	3	0	3	7	18	36	175	2	High in calories.
Apple butter	1 tablespoon (0.6 oz.)	0	0	0	0	1	1	1	0	2	33	1	Has 30% fewer calories than jelly.
Apple pie	4" sector of 9" diam. pie (4.8 oz.)	4	4	2	1	1	1	5	36	117	330	1	Most pies are high in calories.
Apricot: Fresh	1 apricot (1.3 oz.)	0	19	1	1	1	1	2	0	0	18	22	Wonderful for vitamin A.
Canned with syrup	4 halves with syrup (4.3 oz.)	0	43	1	2	0	1	4	0	2	105	8	The syrup increases the calories.
Dried, uncooked	10 small halves (1.3 oz.)	3	82	0	3	6	3	20	0	2	98	19	Outstanding in vitamin A.
Apricot nectar	1/2 cup (4 fl. oz.)	0	24	1	1	5	0	2	0	2	70	8	
Arrowroot starch	1 tablespoon (0.3 oz.)	0	0	0	0	0	0	0	0	2	30	0	
Asparagus: Green spears	6 medium (3.4 oz.)	3	15	4	4	23	2	18	0	2	20	55	Excellent for reducing diets.
Bleached spears	6 medium (3.4 oz.)	3	1	3	4	23	2	10	0	2	20	36	Note how bleaching reduces vitamin A.
Asparagus cream soup	1 cup (8 fl. oz.)	10	4	3	11	4	27	5	63	108	200	4	
Avocado	1/2 avocado (3.8 oz.)	3	6	8	12	20	1	6	36	162	185	5	Low in saturated fat.
Bacon: Cooked crisp and drained	2 slices (0.6 oz.)	7	0	3	3	0	1	5	27	72	95	2	Cook very crisp to reduce the fat.
Canadian, broiled or fried	1 slice (1 oz.)	21	0	16	3	0	1	12	21	45	79	7	Much lower in fat than regular bacon.
Banana	1 medium (5.3 oz.)	1	4	3	3	13	1	7	0	2	85	6	Preferable to candy for between-meal snacks.
Barley, light, pearled, cooked	1/2 cup (4-1/2 oz.)	4	0	2	2	0	1	7	0	2	121	2	
Barley soup	1 cup (8 fl. oz.)	9	1	1	3	0	10	2	9	36	115	2	
Beans: Common varieties with sauce	1/2 cup (4.6 oz.)	11	1	4	3	3	11	26	4	4	158	5	
Pork and beans with sauce	1/2 cup (4.6 oz.)	11	1	4	3	3	11	22	14	32	165	4	Rich in iron, protein, and vitamin B_1.
Garbanzo beans, cooked	1/2 cup (2.8 oz.)	11	0	10	4	0	4	27	3	16	138	5	
Lima, baby, cooked	1/2 cup (2.8 oz.)	6	5	7	4	16	3	14	0	4	75	11	
Lima, dried, cooked	1/2 cup (3.4 oz.)	11	0	8	3	0	4	28	0	4	130	6	
Red kidney or navy beans, cooked	1/2 cup (4.5 oz.)	11	0	4	4	0	5	23	0	4	115	5	
Soybeans, green, cooked	1/2 cup (2.8 oz.)	11	11	16	6	18	6	20	7	37	94	14	Contains complete protein – high in desirable fat.
Soybeans, dried, cooked	1/2 cup (2.8 oz.)	16	1	14	6	0	9	26	11	53	107	9	
Beans, string or snap: Green beans cooked fast, little water	1/2 cup (2.2 oz.)	1	8	3	3	12	3	4	0	1	14	39	Fine for reducing diets.
cooked slowly, much water	1/2 cup (2.2 oz.)	1	8	2	3	8	3	4	0	1	14	33	Note how overcooking can reduce vitamin C.

HEALTH-BUILDING VALUES OF FOODS

FOOD	AMOUNT	PROTEIN	Vitamin A	Vitamin B₁	Vitamin B₂	Vitamin C	Calcium	Iron	Saturated Fat Calories	Total Fat Calories (Both saturated and unsaturated)	TOTAL CALORIES (from protein, fat, and carbohydrate)	V-M INDEX	REMARKS (The Vitamin-Mineral Index is shown at left. The higher the Index number, the more vitamins and minerals per calorie of food.)
Green beans, canned	1/2 cup with liquid (4.2 oz.)	1	10	2	3	6	4	16	0	1	22	31	
Wax or yellow snap beans, canned	1/2 cup with liquid (4.2 oz.)	2	2	2	3	6	4	16	0	1	22	25	Note lower vitamin A content of yellow beans.
Bean soup	1 cup (8 fl. oz.)	11	0	6	6	0	12	28	18	45	190	5	
Bean sprouts: Mung beans	1/2 cup (1.6 oz.)	2	0	2	6	9	2	4	0	1	10	32	A crunchy addition to salads –delicious when steamed.
Soybean sprouts	1/2 cup (1.9 oz.)	5	2	8	6	9	3	6	1	4	25	23	A delicious food for modern low calorie meals.
Beef, cooked:													
Hamburger broiled (market ground)	1 medium patty (3 oz.)	30	1	4	1	0	1	27	72	153	245	2	62% of the calories are from fat.
Hamburger broiled (ground lean)	1 medium patty (3 oz.)	33	0	5	11	0	1	30	45	90	185	4	
Hamburger with bun	One (meat 1.5 oz., bun 1.8 oz.)	21	0	10	7	0	6	27	44	97	254	3	
Heart, braised (fat trimmed)	1 piece (3 oz.)	37	1	14	58	4	2	59	18	45	160	14	High in protein, B complex vitamins, and iron.
Kidneys, cooked	1 piece (3 oz.)	35	38	30	230	28	2	128	60	119	230	33	Rich in protein, B complex vitamins, and iron.
Liver, fried	1 piece (3 oz.)	28	910	14	188	36	1	66	27	54	180	112	Outstanding in protein, vitamins, and minerals.
Liver, calf, fried	1 piece (3 oz.)	28	466	11	175	40	1	106	45	91	184	72	Liver is one of the most nutritious foods you can eat.
Roast, fatty cut such as rib	3 slices 1/4"x2-1/4"x2-3/4" (3 oz.)	23	1	2	7	0	1	21	153	324	390	1	83% of the calories are fat calories.
Roast, fatty cut (outside fat trimmed)	3 slices (3 oz.)	33	1	4	10	0	1	30	45	105	200	4	Modern folks trim the fat for improved nutrition.
Roast, lean cut such as round	3 slices 1/4"x2-1/4"x2-3/4" (3 oz.)	33	1	4	10	0	1	32	63	126	220	3	
Roast, lean cut (outside fat trimmed)	3 slices (3 oz.)	36	0	4	11	0	1	32	22	43	156	5	Trimming fat reduces saturated fat.
Roast, veal	3 oz.	33	1	7	14	0	1	29	63	126	305	2	74% of the calories are from fat.
Steak, fatty cut such as sirloin	1 slice 1"x2"x3-1/2" (3 oz.)	29	1	3	9	0	1	25	117	243	330	2	
Steak, fatty cut (outside fat trimmed)	1 slice (3 oz.)	37	0	4	11	0	1	31	26	51	165	5	Notice the decrease in fat calories when trimmed.
Steak, lean cut such as round	1 slice 1/2"x2"x2-1/2" (3 oz.)	34	0	4	11	0	1	30	54	117	220	3	Leaner meats contain more protein.
Steak, lean cut (outside fat trimmed)	1 slice (3 oz.)	39	0	4	11	0	1	32	22	44	160	5	Note drop in saturated fat calories.
Veal cutlet, broiled	Without bone (3 oz.)	33	0	4	12	0	1	27	36	81	185	4	
Various cuts	3 oz.	33	0	3	10	0	1	29	72	144	245	4	
Various cuts (outside fat trimmed)	3 oz.	37	0	3	11	0	1	32	20	53	165	5	Trimming off fat may help your arteries.
Beef products: Beef and vegetable stew	1 cup (8.3 oz.)	21	51	8	10	19	4	28	45	90	185	11	
Beef soup	1 cup (8 fl. oz.)	9	0	0	0	0	0	5	18	36	100	1	Excellent for modern low calorie meals.
Bouillon	1 cup (8 fl. oz.)	3	0	0	3	0	0	10	0	0	10	22	
Chipped beef, dried	2 oz.	27	0	2	10	0	1	29	18	36	115	6	
Corned beef, canned	3 oz.	31	0	2	11	0	2	37	45	90	180	5	
Corned beef hash	3 oz.	17	0	1	6	0	3	11	18	45	120	3	
Potpie, baked	1 pie 4-1/2" diam. (8 oz.)	26	57	4	8	0	2	25	90	252	460	3	
Beer	12 fl. oz.	2	0	0	8	0	2	0	0	0	171	1	
Beets: Cooked, diced	1/2 cup (2.9 oz.)	1	0	1	2	7	2	6	0	3	35	9	
Greens, cooked	1/2 cup (2.6 oz.)	2	108	2	6	15	2	23	0	0	20	128	Outstanding in vitamins and minerals – low in calories.
Biscuits, enriched flour	1 biscuit 2-1/2" diam. (1.3 oz.)	4	0	6	5	0	8	7	9	36	130	3	
Blackberries, fresh	1/2 cup (2.5 oz.)	1	3	2	5	20	3	6	0	4	42	14	

HEALTH-BUILDING VALUES OF FOODS

FOOD	AMOUNT	% OF DAILY ALLOWANCE							Saturated Fat Calories	Total Fat Calories (Both saturated and unsaturated)	TOTAL CALORIES (From protein, fat, and carbohydrate)	V-M INDEX	REMARKS (The Vitamin-Mineral Index is shown at left. The higher the Index number, the more vitamins and minerals per calorie of food.)
		PROTEIN	Vitamin A	Vitamin B$_1$	Vitamin B$_2$	Vitamin C	Calcium	Iron					
Blackeyed peas	1/2 cup (4.4 oz.)	9	0	13	3	-0	3	16	0	4	95	6	
Blackstrap molasses	1 tablespoon (0.7 oz.)	0	0	1	2	0	14	23	0	0	45	15	This food is an excellent natural laxative.
Blanc mange	1/2 cup (4.4 oz.)	6	4	2	11	1	18	1	27	45	138	4	
Blue cheese salad dressing	1 tablespoon (0.6 oz.)	1	1	0	1	0	1	0	18	86	90	4	Contains valuable linoleic fat.
Blueberries, fresh	1/2 cup (2.5 oz.)	1	1	1	2	13	1	7	0	4	42	10	
Bluefish, baked or broiled	3 oz.	31	1	6	4	0	3	6	7	36	135	2	Fish are high in protein and low in saturated fat.
Bologna	2 slices 4" diam. (2 oz.)	10	0	6	7	0	1	6	60	140	172	2	High in fat.
Boston brown bread	1 slice (1.7 oz.)	4	0	3	2	0	5	9	0	9	100	3	
Bouillon cubes	One 5/8" cube (0.1 oz.)	0	0	0	0	0	0	0	0	2	2	33	Often used in low calorie diets.
Bouillon soup	1 cup (8 fl. oz.)	3	0	1	3	0	0	10	0	2	10	22	Excellent for modern low calorie meals.
Brains, all kinds, cooked	3 oz.	15	0	12	15	24	2	38	32	80	129	12	High in vitamins and minerals.
Bran: All-bran cereal	1/2 cup (1.1 oz.)	5	0	7	6	0	4	31	1	9	72	11	Rich in iron.
Flakes, 40% bran	1 oz.	3	0	8	4	0	2	11	1	9	85	5	
Raisin-bran cereal	1 cup (1.8 oz.)	6	0	12	5	0	4	24	1	8	149	5	
Brandy, 86 proof	1 jigger (1-1/2 fl. oz.)	0	0	0	0	0	0	0	0	0	108	0	Empty calories.
Brazil nuts	1 tbsp. broken pieces (0.3 oz.)	2	0	5	0	0	2	3	10	52	57	3	Rich in linoleic fat.
Bread: Boston brown bread	1 slice (1.7 oz.)	4	0	3	2	0	5	3	4	9	100	3	
Cornbread with enriched meal	1 piece (1.7 oz.)	6	3	6	8	0	10	4	18	45	155	4	
Cracked wheat	1 slice (0.8 oz.)	3	0	2	1	0	2	3	4	9	60	2	
Pumpernickel, dark	1 slice (0.8 oz.)	3	0	3	2	0	2	6	1	2	56	4	
Raisin bread	1 slice (0.8 oz.)	3	0	1	1	0	2	3	4	9	60	2	
Rye bread, light	1 slice (0.8 oz.)	3	0	2	1	0	2	4	0	4	55	3	
White bread, enriched	1 slice (0.8 oz.)	3	0	4	3	0	3	6	4	9	60	3	
100% Whole wheat	1 slice (0.8 oz.)	3	0	4	3	0	3	5	4	9	55	5	This is the most nutritious bread.
Breadcrumbs	1 tablespoon (0.2 oz.)	1	0	1	1	0	1	2	1	2	22	4	
Broccoli, cooked	1/2 cup (2.6 oz.)	4	51	3	6	74	12	10	1	1	22	118	Excellent for vitamin A and vitamin C.
Brown betty with apple	1/2 cup (4.1 oz.)	3	3	4	3	0	3	7	18	36	175	2	High in calories.
Brussels sprouts, cooked	1/2 cup (2.3 oz.)	4	5	2	4	41	3	8	0	4	30	35	Rich in vitamin C.
Buckwheat flour: Dark	1 cup sifted (3.5 oz.)	16	0	35	8	0	4	27	3	22	340	4	
Light	1 cup sifted (3.5 oz.)	9	0	5	2	0	2	10	3	11	342	1	Refining reduces nutritive values.
Buckwheat pancakes	1 pancake (1 oz.)	3	1	2	2	0	8	3	9	18	45	6	
Buns	1 bun (1.8 oz.)	7	0	2	3	0	3	4	9	18	160	2	
Butter	1 pat (0.2 oz.)	0	5	0	0	0	0	0	27	50	50	1	High in saturated fat.
	1 tablespoon (1/2 oz.)	0	9	0	0	0	0	0	54	100	100	2	
Buttermilk	1 cup (8 fl. oz.)	12	1	6	24	4	36	2	1	2	87	14	Helps you avoid saturated fat.
	1 quart (32 fl. oz.)	49	1	22	97	17	144	7	5	9	348	14	
Butterscotch candy	1 oz.	0	0	0	0	1	1	5	0	22	116	1	

HEALTH-BUILDING VALUES OF FOODS

FOOD	AMOUNT	% OF DAILY ALLOWANCE							Saturated Fat Calories	Total Fat Calories (Both saturated and unsaturated)	TOTAL CALORIES (Plus protein, fat, and carbohydrate)	V-M INDEX	REMARKS (The Vitamin-Mineral Index is shown at left. The higher the Index number, the more vitamins and minerals per calorie of food.)
		PROTEIN	Vitamin A	Vitamin B₁	Vitamin B₂	Vitamin C	Calcium	Iron					
Cabbage: Raw, shredded	1/2 cup (1.8 oz.)	1	1	2	1	33	3	2	0	1	12	58	Good source of roughage and vitamin C.
Quickly cooked, little water	1/2 cup (3 oz.)	1	1	2	1	35	5	4	0	1	20	42	Excellent for modern low calorie meals.
Slowly cooked, much water	1/2 cup (3 oz.)	1	2	2	1	21	5	4	0	1	20	29	Prolonged cooking reduces vitamin C.
Coleslaw made with dressing	1/2 cup (2.1 oz.)	1	1	0	1	33	3	2	4	32	50	14	
Cake: Angel food cake	2" sector of 8" diam. cake (1.4 oz.)	4	0	0	3	0	3	1	0	2	110	1	
Chocolate cake with fudge icing	2" sector of 8" diam. cake (4.2 oz.)	7	3	2	6	0	15	5	45	126	420	1	Very high in calories.
Cupcake without icing	1 cupcake 2-3/4" diam. (1.8 oz.)	4	1	2	2	0	7	2	9	27	160	1	Cake calories do not help achieve optimal nutrition.
Fruitcake	2" square x 1/2" thick (1.1 oz.)	3	1	2	2	0	4	8	9	36	105	3	
Gingerbread	2" cube (1.9 oz.)	3	1	1	3	0	8	14	18	63	180	2	
Layer cake with icing	2" sector of 10" diam. cake (3.5 oz.)	7	2	1	4	0	15	4	18	54	320	1	
Plain cake without icing	3" x 2" x 1-1/2" (1.9 oz.)	6	1	1	3	0	11	2	9	45	180	2	
Pound cake	2-3/4" x 3" x 5/8" (1.1 oz.)	3	2	1	3	0	2	5	18	63	130	2	
Sponge cake	2" sector of 8" diam. cake (1.4 oz.)	4	1	1	3	0	6	6	9	18	115	2	
Calf liver, fried	1 piece (3 oz.)	28	466	11	175	40	1	106	45	91	184	72	Liver is one of the most nutritious foods you can eat.
Canadian bacon, broiled or fried	1 piece (1 oz.)	11	0	16	3	0	1	12	21	45	79	7	Much lower than regular bacon in total fat.
Candy: Butterscotch	1 oz.	0	0	0	0	0	1	5	0	22	116	1	
Candied citron, grapefruit, lemon or orange peel	1 oz.	0	0	0	0	0	3	2	0	1	89	1	
Candied ginger root	1 oz.	0	0	0	0	0	0	7	0	1	97	0	
Caramels	1 oz.	1	1	1	2	0	4	7	18	27	120	2	Candies that stick between teeth hasten decay.
Chocolate creams	1 oz.	2	0	0	0	0	0	0	20	36	110	0	Watch that bulging figure!
Fondant	1 oz.	0	0	0	0	0	0	0	0	0	101	1	Almost pure sugar.
Fudge	1 oz.	0	1	0	1	0	2	1	18	27	115	0	Delicious – but not for modern low calorie diets.
Hard candy	1 oz.	0	0	0	0	0	0	0	0	0	110	1	Empty calories.
Marshmallow	1 oz.	1	0	1	2	0	0	0	0	0	90	0	Dentists deplore these relatively empty calories.
Milk chocolate	1 oz.	3	1	2	6	0	8	3	45	81	145	2	
Peanut brittle	1 oz.	1	0	4	4	0	1	6	9	40	125		
Cantaloupe	1/2 melon (13.6 oz.)	1	132	6	4	84	4	4	0	2	40	99	Fine for vitamins A and C – low in calories.
Carrot: Raw	1 carrot 5-1/2" long (1.8 oz.)	1	120	2	2	4	2	4	0	2	20	112	High in vitamin A.
Raw, grated	1/2 cup (1.9 oz.)	1	132	2	2	5	3	4	0	2	22	112	
Cooked, diced	1/2 cup (2.6 oz.)	1	181	2	4	4	0	4	0	4	22	148	The vitamin A is more available after cooking.
Cashew nuts, roasted	1 tablespoon (0.3 oz.)	2	0	2	2	0	0	3	6	37	48	2	
Cauliflower, cooked	1/2 cup (2.1 oz.)	2	0	1	3	23	2	6	0	1	15	41	Excellent for modern low calorie meals.
Celery: Raw	1 stalk 8" long (1.4 oz.)	1	1	1	1	4	2	2	0	1	7	24	Low in calories – excellent for roughage.
Raw, diced	1/2 cup (1.8 oz.)	1	0	0	2	5	3	2	0	1	9	24	
Celery cream soup	1 cup (8 fl. oz.)	10	4	3	11	0	27	5	63	108	200	4	
Cereals: All-bran	1/2 cup (1.1 oz.)	5	0	7	6	0	4	31	1	9	72	11	Rich in iron.

HEALTH-BUILDING VALUES OF FOODS

FOOD	AMOUNT	PROTEIN	Vitamin A	Vitamin B₁	Vitamin B₂	Vitamin C	Calcium	Iron	Saturated Fat Calories	Total Fat Calories (Both saturated and unsaturated)	TOTAL CALORIES (From protein, fat, and carbohydrate)	V-M INDEX	REMARKS (The Vitamin-Mineral Index is shown at left. The higher the Index number, the more vitamins and minerals per calorie of food.)
Cereals: Bran flakes, 40% bran	1 oz.	4	0	8	4	0	2	11	1	9	85	5	
Bran, Raisin bran	1 cup (1.8 oz.)	6	0	12	5	0	4	24	1	8	149	5	
Corn flakes	1 oz.	3	0	8	2	0	0	5	0	2	110	2	
Corn flakes, sweetened	1 oz.	1	0	8	1	0	0	4	0	2	110	2	
Corn and soy shreds	1 oz.	7	0	12	2	0	3	12	0	2	100	5	
Farina, cooked, enriched	1/2 cup (4.2 oz.)	2	0	3	2	0	2	2	0	1	52	4	
Oat cereal mixture, enriched	1 oz.	6	0	14	2	0	6	12	4	18	115	5	
Oatmeal or rolled oats	1/2 cup (4.2 oz.)	4	0	7	1	0	1	8	4	14	75	4	
Rice flakes	1 cup (1.1 oz.)	3	0	4	1	0	1	5	0	2	115	2	
Rice, puffed	1 cup (1/2 oz.)	1	0	4	1	0	0	3	0	2	55	2	
Wheat flakes, enriched	1 oz.	4	0	10	3	0	2	12	0	2	100	5	
Wheat germ	1/2 cup stirred (1.2 oz.)	12	0	43	15	0	4	28	4	32	123	12	By far the most nutritious cereal – contains complete protein.
Wheat, puffed, enriched	1 oz.	6	0	10	3	0	1	12	0	2	100	4	
Wheat, puffed, sweetened, enriched	1 oz.	1	0	8	1	0	1	5	0	2	105	2	
Wheat, shredded	1 oz.	4	0	4	2	0	2	10	0	9	100	3	
Wheat and malted barley, enriched	1 oz.	4	0	8	3	0	0	10	0	2	105	4	
Champagne	1 glass (3 oz.)	0	0	0	0	0	0	2	0	0	75	0	
Cheese: Cheddar or American	1" cube (0.6 oz.)	6	5	0	4	0	17	0	27	54	70	7	High in fat calories.
Cheddar or American, grated	1 tablespoon (0.2 oz.)	3	2	1	2	0	7	1	9	18	30	7	
Cheddar, process	1 oz.	10	7	0	7	0	27	2	45	81	105	7	
Cheese spreads, Cheddar	1 oz.	9	6	1	9	0	20	2	36	63	95	7	
Cottage cheese, uncreamed	1/2 cup (4 oz.)	27	0	2	18	0	13	4	1	4	98	6	Blend with a little whole milk to improve taste.
Cottage cheese, creamed	1/2 cup (4 oz.)	21	4	2	18	0	13	4	27	50	120	6	
Cream cheese	1 tablespoon (1/2 oz.)	1	4	0	1	0	1	0	27	52	55	2	Almost all the calories are fat calories.
Limburger	1 piece (1 oz.)	9	7	1	8	0	21	2	39	71	97	7	
Parmesan	1 piece (1 oz.)	15	6	1	12	0	41	1	37	67	112	9	High in calcium.
Roquefort	1 oz.	9	7	1	9	0	15	1	45	81	105	5	High in saturated fat.
Swiss	1 oz.	10	6	1	3	0	34	3	36	72	105	7	Note saturated fat calories.
Cherries: Fresh, sour, sweet, or hybrid	1/2 cup (2 oz.)	1	6	2	2	6	2	2	0	4	32	10	
Red, canned	1/2 cup (4.4 oz.)	1	17	2	2	9	2	4	0	4	52	12	
Surinam cherry	3.5 oz.	1	30	2	2	40	1	2	0	4	51	25	Good for vitamins A and C.
Cherry pie	4" sector of 9" diam. pie (4.8 oz.)	4	10	2	2	3	1	5	36	117	340	3	
Chicken: Broiled	Without bone (3 oz.)	33	5	2	8	0	1	14	27	81	185	3	Has less saturated fat than beef or pork.
Fried breast	1/2 breast with bone (3.3 oz.)	34	1	2	3	0	1	11	27	108	215	1	
Fried leg and thigh	With bone (4.3 oz.)	39	4	3	10	0	2	18	36	135	245	3	
Canned, boneless	3 oz.	36	3	2	8	0	2	15	18	63	170	3	

% OF DAILY ALLOWANCE

HEALTH-BUILDING VALUES OF FOODS

FOOD	AMOUNT	PROTEIN	Vitamin A	Vitamin B_1	Vitamin B_2	Vitamin C	Calcium	Iron	Saturated Fat Calories	Total Fat Calories (Both saturated and unsaturated)	TOTAL CALORIES (From protein, fat, and carbohydrate)	V-M INDEX	REMARKS (The Vitamin-Mineral Index is shown at left. The higher the Index number, the more vitamins and minerals per calorie of food.)
				% OF DAILY ALLOWANCE									
Chicken: Liver, fried	3 chicken livers (3 oz.)	32	667	11	139	23	2	74	24	74	184	83	Liver contains nutrients not yet identified.
Chicken potpie	1 pie, 4-1/2" diam. (8 oz.)	24	37	4	8	0	5	16	72	252	485	2	
Chicken soup	1 cup (8 fl. oz.)	6	0	1	7	0	5	5	9	18	75	3	
Chickpeas, cooked	1/2 cup (2.8 oz.)	11	0	10	4	0	4	27	3	16	138	5	Rich in iron, protein, and vitamin B_1.
Chile con carne: With beans	1 cup (8.8 oz.)	27	3	5	4	0	12	42	63	135	335	4	
Without beans	1 cup (9 oz.)	37	8	3	17	0	12	36	162	342	510	2	
Chili powder	1 teaspoon (0.2 oz.)	1	77	1	4	1	1	4	0	3	17	86	
Chili sauce	1 tablespoon (0.6 oz.)	0	6	1	1	3	1	4	0	2	15	13	
Chipped beef, dried	2 oz.	27	0	1	10	0	1	29	18	36	115	6	
Chocolate: Unsweetened	1 oz.	3	0	1	3	0	4	12	72	135	145	2	High in fat calories.
Sweetened	1 oz.	1	0	2	2	0	15	8	27	72	135	1	
Chocolate cake with fudge icing	2" sector of 8" diam. cake (4.2 oz.)	7	3	2	6	0	15	8	45	126	420	2	Very high in calories.
Chocolate candy, milk chocolate	1 oz.	3	1	2	6	0	8	3	45	81	145	0	
Chocolate cream candy	1 oz.	2	0	0	0	0	3	3	20	36	110	6	Watch that bulging figure!
Chocolate milk	1 cup (8 fl. oz.)	11	4	6	23	3	34	4	27	54	190	1	
Chocolate syrup	1 tablespoon (0.7 oz.)	0	0	0	0	0	0	1	1	2	42	2	
Chop: Lamb, broiled	1 chop (4 oz.)	36	0	9	14	0	0	31	162	297	405	5	
Lamb, broiled (fat trimmed)	1 chop (2.6 oz.)	30	0	7	11	0	1	25	27	54	140	5	Trimming helps you lower your fat total.
Pork, cooked	1 chop (3-1/2 oz.)	23	0	39	10	0	1	22	72	189	260	8	
Pork, cooked (fat trimmed)	1 chop (1.7 oz.)	21	0	34	9	0	1	19	27	63	130	20	Calories cut in half when fat trimmed - other nutrients largely unchanged.
Clams: Raw	Without shell (3 oz.)	16	2	5	8	0	10	60	2	9	70	26	Clams are very high in iron.
Canned	With liquid (3 oz.)	10	1	2	4	0	9	54	2	9	45	8	
Clam chowder	1 cup (8 fl. oz.)	7	0	4	2	0	4	36	2	18	85	9	
Cocoa: Dry powder	1 tablespoon (0.2 oz.)	1	0	1	25	3	36	9	9	15	21	6	
Made with milk	1 cup (8 fl. oz.)	13	8	6	25	3	36	9	54	99	235	1	
Coconut: Fresh, shredded	1 tablespoon (0.2 oz.)	0	0	6	0	0	0	1	15	17	21	1	
Dried, shredded, sweetened	1 tablespoon (0.1 oz.)	0	0	1	0	0	0	1	12	14	22	31	
Cod liver oil, U.S.P.	1 tablespoon (1/2 oz.)	0	255	0	0	0	0	0	20	135	135	3	A tablespoon also contains 1,275 units of vitamin D.
Codfish, cooked	3 oz.	25	0	3	5	0	1	5	1	4	79	0	Ocean fish are rich in iodine and trace minerals.
Coffee, without sugar or cream	1 cup (8 fl. oz.)	0	0	0	0	0	0	0	0	0	0	0	
Cola type drink	1 cup (8 fl. oz.)	0	0	0	0	0	0	0	0	0	105	0	Dentists deplore these empty calories.
Coleslaw	1/2 cup (2.1 oz.)	1	1	2	1	33	3	0	0	32	50	14	
Collards, cooked	1/2 cup (3.4 oz.)	5	145	5	13	56	30	15	0	4	38	116	High in vitamins A, C, and minerals - low in calories.
Condensed milk, sweetened	1 tablespoon (0.7 oz.)	2	1	1	3	0	6	0	8	14	62	3	
Consommé	1 cup (8 fl. oz.)	3	0	0	0	0	0	10	0	0	10	22	Excellent for modern low calorie meals.
Cookies: Assorted kinds	One 3" cookie (0.9 oz.)	3	0	1	1	0	1	2	9	27	110	1	Rather empty calories.

HEALTH-BUILDING VALUES OF FOODS

FOOD	AMOUNT	PROTEIN	Vitamin A	Vitamin B₁	Vitamin B₂	Vitamin C	Calcium	Iron	Saturated Fat Calories	Total Fat Calorie (Both saturated and unsaturated)	TOTAL CALORIES (From protein, fat, and carbohydrate)	V-M INDEX	REMARKS (The Vitamin-Mineral Index is shown at left. The higher the Index number, the more vitamins and minerals per calorie of food.)
Cookies: Fig bars	1 small bar (0.6 oz.)	1	0	0	1	0	1	2	4	9	55	1	
Cooking oil: Corn oil	1 tablespoon (1/2 oz.)	0	0	0	0	0	0	0	18	125	125	0	Rich in desirable unsaturated linoleic fat.
Cottonseed oil	1 tablespoon (1/2 oz.)	0	0	0	0	0	0	0	27	125	125	0	Rich in desirable unsaturated linoleic fat.
Olive oil	1 tablespoon (1/2 oz.)	0	0	0	0	0	0	0	18	125	125	0	Rich in unsaturated fat - though low in linoleic fat.
Soybean oil	1 tablespoon (1/2 oz.)	0	0	0	0	0	0	0	18	125	125	0	High in helpful linoleic fat.
Cordials and liqueurs, 80 proof	1 jigger (1-1/2 oz.)	0	0	0	0	0	1	0	0	0	146	0	
Corn: Cooked	One 5" ear (4.9 oz.)	3	6	6	4	8	1	5	1	9	65	8	
Canned	1/2 cup (4.5 oz.)	4	5	2	4	9	1	6	0	4	85	5	
Corn bread, enriched corn meal	1 piece (1.7 oz.)	6	3	6	8	0	10	9	18	45	155	4	
Corn cereals: Corn and soy shreds	1 oz.	7	0	12	2	0	3	12	0	2	100	5	
Flakes, enriched	1 oz.	3	0	8	1	0	0	5	0	2	110	2	
Flakes, sweetened, enriched	1 oz.	1	0	8	3	0	0	4	0	2	110	2	
Puffed, sweetened	1 oz.	1	0	8	0	0	0	5	0	2	110	2	
Corn grits, white, cooked, enriched	1/2 cup (4.3 oz.)	2	0	3	0	0	0	4	0	1	60	3	
Corn meal: Dry whole ground	1/2 cup (2.1 oz.)	8	6	14	4	0	1	14	4	22	210	3	
Dry, degermed, enriched	1/2 cup (2.6 oz.)	8	4	20	11	0	1	21	4	9	262	4	
Corn muffins made with enriched meal	1 muffin (1.7 oz.)	6	3	6	8	0	10	9	18	45	155	4	Rich in desirable unsaturated linoleic fat.
Corn oil	1 tablespoon (1/2 oz.)	0	0	0	0	0	0	0	18	125	125	0	
Cornstarch	1 tablespoon (0.3 oz.)	0	0	0	0	0	0	0	0	2	30	0	
Cornstarch pudding (Blanc mange)	1/2 cup (4.4 oz.)	6	4	2	11	1	18	1	27	45	138	4	
Corned beef, canned	3 oz.	31	0	1	11	0	2	37	45	90	180	5	
Corned beef hash	3 oz.	17	0	1	6	0	3	11	18	45	120	3	
Cottage cheese: Uncreamed	1/2 cup (4 oz.)	27	0	2	18	0	13	4	1	4	98	6	Blend with a little whole milk to improve taste.
Creamed	1/2 cup (4 oz.)	21	4	2	18	0	13	4	27	50	120	6	
Cottonseed oil	1 tablespoon (1/2 oz.)	0	0	0	0	0	0	0	27	125	125	0	Rich in desirable unsaturated linoleic fat.
Cowpeas, cooked	1/2 cup (4.4 oz.)	9	0	13	3	0	3	16	4	4	95	6	
Crabmeat, canned or cooked	3 oz.	20	0	2	3	0	5	8	4	18	90	3	
Cracked wheat bread	1 slice (0.8 oz.)	3	0	2	1	0	1	3	4	9	60	2	
Crackers: Graham	4 small or 2 medium (1/2 oz.)	1	0	2	1	0	1	3	4	9	55	2	
Oyster crackers	10 crackers (0.4 oz.)	1	0	1	0	0	0	1	4	9	45	1	
Ry-Krisp type	2 wafers about 2"x3" (1/2 oz.)	3	0	2	2	0	1	6	0	2	42	4	Most crackers are high in calories - low in other values.
Saltines	2 crackers 2" square (0.3 oz.)	1	0	1	0	0	0	1	4	9	35	0	
Soda crackers	2 crackers 2-1/2" square (0.4 oz.)	1	0	1	1	0	0	1	4	9	45	1	
Cracker bread	1 tablespoon (0.4 oz.)	1	0	1	0	0	1	2	4	9	45	1	
Cranberry juice	1/2 cup (4.4 oz.)	0	0	0	1	3	1	1	0	1	70	2	
Cranberry sauce	1 tablespoon (0.6 oz.)	0	0	0	0	0	0	0	0	1	34	1	
Cream: Half milk, half cream	1 tablespoon (1/2 oz.)	0	1	0	1	0	2	0	9	18	20	3	

HEALTH-BUILDING VALUES OF FOODS

FOOD	AMOUNT	PROTEIN	Vitamin A	Vitamin B_1	Vitamin B_2	Vitamin C	Calcium	Iron	Saturated Fat Calories	Total Fat Calories (Both saturated and unsaturated)	TOTAL CALORIES (From protein, fat, and carbohydrate)	V-M INDEX	REMARKS (The Vitamin-Mineral Index is shown at left. The higher the Index number, the more vitamins and minerals per calorie of food.)
Cream: Light cream	1 tablespoon (1/2 oz.)	0	3	0	1	0	2	0	18	27	35	3	Mainly fat calories.
Medium cream	1 tablespoon (1/2 oz.)	0	4	0	1	0	2	0	27	45	45	3	This runs up your fat total.
Heavy cream	1 tablespoon (1/2 oz.)	0	5	0	1	0	1	0	27	54	55	3	High in undesirable saturated fat.
Whipped, from medium cream	2 tablespoons (1/2 oz.)	0	4	0	1	0	2	0	24	44	45	3	Runs up your fat total.
Whipped, from heavy cream	2 tablespoons (1/2 oz.)	0	5	0	1	0	1	0	29	52	55	2	High in saturated fat.
Cream cheese	1 tablespoon (1/2 oz.)	1	5	0	2	0	1	0	27	52	55	2	Almost all the calories are fat calories.
Cream soups, such as asparagus, celery, mushroom	1 cup (8 fl. oz.)	10	4	3	11	0	27	5	63	108	200	6	
Cress, water	1 oz.	1	27	1	2	29	7	6	0	0	5	240	A good source of vitamins A and C—very few calories.
Cucumber	6 slices (1.8 oz.)	0	0	1	1	5	2	2	0	2	6	28	
Cupcake without icing	1 cupcake 2-3/4" diam. (1.8 oz.)	4	1	1	2	0	7	2	9	27	160	1	Cake calories do not help achieve optimal nutrition.
Currants	1/2 cup (1.9 oz.)	1	1	1	0	27	2	5	0	1	30	20	Fair in vitamin C.
Custard, baked	1/2 cup (4.4 oz.)	9	9	3	13	1	17	5	27	63	142	6	
Custard pie	4" sector of 9" diam. pie (4.6 oz.)	10	6	4	12	0	20	16	36	99	265	4	
Daiquiri cocktail	1 cocktail	0	0	1	0	11	1	1	0	0	124	2	
Dandelion greens, cooked	1/2 cup (3.2 oz.)	4	273	7	6	19	21	28	0	4	40	148	Extremely high in vitamin A, other vitamins, & minerals.
Dates, pitted	4 dates (1 oz.)	1	1	2	2	0	3	9	0	4	81	3	
Doughnuts	1 doughnut (1.1 oz.)	3	1	3	2	0	3	4	18	63	135	2	
Eels, cooked	3 oz.	31	42	13	24	0	2	8	22	95	188	8	
Eggs: Raw or hard-boiled	1 large egg (1.8 oz.)	9	12	3	8	0	3	11	18	54	80	8	
White of egg	1 egg white (1.2 oz.)	6	0	0	5	0	0	3	0	0	15	6	
Yolk of egg	1 egg yolk (0.6 oz.)	4	12	2	4	0	3	9	18	45	60	8	
Scrambled with milk and fat	1 egg (2.3 oz.)	10	14	3	10	0	6	11	27	72	110	7	Best if scrambled in vegetable oil.
Eggplant, boiled	1/2 cup (3.2 oz.)	1	0	3	2	4	1	5	0	2	17	15	
Endive or escarole	2 oz.	1	34	2	4	8	6	10	0	2	11	97	
Farina, cooked, enriched	1/2 cup (4.2 oz.)	2	0	3	0	0	2	4	0	1	52	4	
Fats: Lard	1 tablespoon (1/2 oz.)	0	0	0	0	0	0	0	45	126	126	0	
Vegetable fats or oils	1 tablespoon (0.4 oz.)	0	0	0	0	0	0	0	27	110	110	0	
Fig newton cookies	1 cookie (0.6 oz.)	1	0	0	1	0	1	2	4	9	55	1	
Figs: Fresh	3 small figs (4 oz.)	3	2	4	3	3	8	7	0	2	90	5	
Dried	1 large fig (0.7 oz.)	1	0	1	1	0	5	7	0	2	60	4	
Fish and shellfish: Bluefish, baked or broiled	3 oz.	31	1	6	4	0	3	6	7	36	135	2	Fish are high in protein and low in saturated fat.
Clams, canned	With liquid (3 oz.)	10	1	2	4	0	9	54	2	9	45	26	Clams are very high in iron.
Clams, raw	Without shell (3 oz.)	16	2	5	8	0	10	9	2	9	70	20	
Cod, cooked	3 oz.	25	0	3	5	0	1	5	1	4	79	3	Ocean fish are rich in iodine and trace minerals.
Crabmeat, cooked	3 oz.	20	0	2	3	0	5	8	4	18	90	3	

HEALTH-BUILDING VALUES OF FOODS

FOOD	AMOUNT	PROTEIN	% OF DAILY ALLOWANCE						Saturated Fat Calories	Total Fat Calories (Both saturated and unsaturated)	TOTAL CALORIES (From protein, fat, and carbohydrate)	V-M INDEX	REMARKS (The Vitamin-Mineral Index is shown at left. The higher the Index number, the more vitamins and minerals per calorie of food.)
			Vitamin A	Vitamin B1	Vitamin B2	Vitamin C	Calcium	Iron					
Fish and shellfish: Eels, cooked	3 oz.	31	42	13	24	0	2	8	22	95	188	8	
Fishsticks, breaded	4 sticks 1/2"x1"x3-3/4" (3.2 oz.)	21	1	2	3	0	1	4	18	72	160	1	Rich in minerals from the ocean.
Haddock, fried	3 oz.	23	1	2	4	0	1	5	9	45	135	2	Contains vitamin D which is scarce in foods grown in soil.
Halibut, broiled	3 oz.	32	7	2	3	0	2	7	12	60	155	2	
Herring, smoked, kippered	3 oz.	27	0	0	13	0	7	12	18	99	180	3	Low in saturated fat.
Lobster, canned	3 oz.	22	9	2	3	0	7	7	2	10	78	4	High quality protein with little fat.
Mackerel, broiled	3 oz.	27	9	8	13	0	1	10	23	117	200	3	Fish are ideal for modern diets.
Ocean perch, breaded and fried	3 oz.	23	1	6	6	0	2	13	20	99	195	2	Complete protein with low fat content - rich in iron.
Oysters, raw without shell	1/2 cup, about 8 med. (4.2 oz.)	14	7	9	11	0	14	66	4	18	80	22	
Oyster stew with milk	1 cup, 3 to 4 oysters (8 fl. oz.)	16	13	8	22	9	34	33	22	108	200	9	Contains the elusive vitamin D.
Salmon, canned	3 oz.	24	4	1	9	0	20	7	9	45	120	5	Rich in protein, minerals, and a desirable type of fat.
Sardines, canned in oil and drained	3 oz.	31	4	1	10	0	46	25	18	81	180	8	Top quality protein with practically no fat.
Scallops, cooked	3 oz.	30	0	3	8	0	4	5	0	1	109	8	
Shad, baked	3 oz.	29	0	7	12	0	2	5	18	90	170	3	
Shrimp, canned	3 oz.	33	1	1	2	0	12	26	2	9	110	6	High in protein – low in fat.
Swordfish, broiled with butter or margarine	3 oz.	34	35	2	2	0	3	11	9	45	150	6	
Tuna, canned in oil, and drained	3 oz.	36	1	2	6	0	1	12	18	63	170	6	One of the few foods with a worthwhile amt. of vit. D.
Fishsticks, breaded	4 sticks 1/2"x1"x3-3/4" (3.2 oz.)	21	0	2	3	0	1	4	18	72	160	1	
Flour: Whole wheat	1 cup (4.2 oz.)	23	0	41	8	0	6	40	3	18	400	4	Note the higher values in whole wheat flour.
White flour, enriched	1 cup sifted (3.9 oz.)	17	0	30	16	0	2	32	1	9	400	3	
White flour, unenriched	1 cup sifted (3.9 oz.)	17	0	8	3	0	2	9	1	9	400	1	
White flour, self-rising, enriched	1 cup (3.9 oz.)	14	0	30	16	0	37	32	1	9	385	5	
White flour, self-rising, unenriched	1 cup (3.9 oz.)	14	0	5	3	0	37	11	1	9	385	1	Refining reduces nutritive values.
Buckwheat flour, light	1 cup sifted (3.5 oz.)	9	0	35	2	0	2	10	2	11	342	1	
Buckwheat flour, dark	1 cup sifted (3.5 oz.)	16	0	35	8	0	4	27	3	22	340	4	Adds top quality inexpensive protein to recipes.
Soybean flour	1 cup (3.1 oz.)	53	2	45	17	0	27	114	8	51	232	15	
Fondant candy	1 oz.	0	0	0	0	0	0	0	0	0	101	0	Almost pure sugar.
Frankfurters	1 frankfurter (1.8 oz.)	9	0	5	6	0	3	3	54	126	155	2	Note high amount of fat.
Frankfurter with bun	One (frank 1.8 oz., bun 1.7 oz.)	16	0	7	8	0	3	12	63	144	315	2	
French salad dressing	1 tablespoon (1/2 oz.)	0	0	0	0	0	0	1	9	48	60	0	Good source of desirable linoleic fat.
Frog legs, cooked	1 pair of legs (3 oz.)	25	4	7	15	0	1	11	1	3	78	7	
Fruit cocktail, with syrup	1/2 cup (4.5 oz.)	1	1	1	1	3	1	5	0	3	98	3	
Fruitcake	2" square x 1/2" thick (1.1 oz.)	3	1	2	2	0	4	8	9	36	105	3	
Fudge candy	1 oz.	0	0	0	1	0	2	1	18	27	115	1	Delicious-but has no place in modern low calorie diets.
Garbanzo beans, cooked	1/2 cup (2.8 oz.)	11	0	10	4	0	4	27	3	16	138	5	Rich in iron, protein, and vitamin B1.

225

HEALTH-BUILDING VALUES OF FOODS

FOOD	AMOUNT	PROTEIN	Vitamin A	Vitamin B_1	Vitamin B_2	Vitamin C	Calcium	Iron	Saturated Fat Calories	Total Fat Calories (Both saturated and unsaturated)	TOTAL CALORIES (From protein, fat, and carbohydrate)	V-M INDEX	REMARKS (The Vitamin-Mineral Index is shown at left. The higher the Index number, the more vitamins and minerals per calorie of food.)
Gelatin: Dry, plain	1 tablespoon (0.4 oz.)	13	0	0	0	0	0	0	0	2	35	0	Contains incomplete protein.
Gelatin dessert	1/2 cup (4.2 oz.)	3	0	0	0	0	0	0	0	1	78	0	
Gelatin dessert with fruit	1/2 cup (4.2 oz.)	2	3	2	1	5	1	4	0	1	85	3	
Gin, 94 proof	1 jigger (1-1/2 fl. oz.)	0	0	0	0	0	0	0	0	0	119	0	Empty calories.
Ginger ale	1 cup (8 fl. oz.)	0	0	0	0	0	0	0	0	0	80	0	More empty calories.
Gingerbread	2" cube (1.9 oz.)	3	1	1	3	0	8	14	18	63	180	2	
Goat's milk	1 cup (8 fl. oz.)	11	8	6	15	3	39	0	54	90	165	7	
Graham crackers	4 small or 2 med. (1/2 oz.)	1	0	2	1	0	3	3	4	9	55	2	
Grapefruit: Fresh	1/2 grapefruit 4-1/4" diam. (10.1 oz.)	1	0	3	1	67	3	3	0	2	50	26	One of the best sources of vitamin C.
Fresh, pink or red	1/2 grapefruit 4-1/4" diam. (10.1 oz.)	1	12	3	1	64	3	5	0	2	55	27	Note the vitamin A in pink grapefruit.
Canned with water	1/2 cup (4.2 oz.)	1	0	2	1	48	2	4	0	1	35	24	
Canned with syrup	1/2 cup (4.4 oz.)	1	0	2	1	50	2	4	0	1	85	12	The added sugar increases the calories.
Grapefruit juice: Fresh	1/2 cup (4 fl. oz.)	1	0	2	1	61	1	5	0	1	48	31	Wonderful for vitamin C.
Canned, unsweetened	1/2 cup (4 fl. oz.)	1	0	2	1	56	1	5	0	1	50	16	
Canned, sweetened	1/2 cup (4 fl. oz.)	1	0	2	1	52	1	5	0	1	65	12	
Juice made from frozen concentrate, sweetened	1/2 cup ready to drink (4 fl. oz.)	1	0	2	1	55	1	1	0	1	58	17	
Juice made from powder	1/2 cup ready to drink (4 fl. oz.)	1	0	3	1	61	1	2	0	1	50	22	
Grapes: Fresh varieties w/slip skins	1 cup (5.4 oz.)	1	2	3	1	5	2	2	1	9	70	4	
Fresh varieties w/adherent skins	1 cup (5.6 oz.)	1	3	5	2	9	2	2	1	2	100	5	
Grape juice	1/2 cup (4 fl. oz.)	1	0	3	2	0	2	4	0	1	82	5	
Green beans: Cooked fast, little water	1/2 cup (2.2 oz.)	1	8	3	3	12	2	4	0	1	14	39	Fine for reducing diets.
Cooked slowly, much water	1/2 cup (2.2 oz.)	1	8	3	3	8	3	4	0	1	14	33	Note how overcooking can reduce vitamin C.
Canned	1/2 cup with liquid (4.2 oz.)	1	10	3	3	6	4	16	0	1	22	31	
Griddle cakes made w/enriched flour	One 4" diam. (1 oz.)	3	1	3	3	1	2	3	2	18	60	4	
Grits, corn grits, white, cooked, enriched	1/2 cup (4.3 oz.)	2	0	2	4	0	1	8	0	1	60	3	
Guavas, fresh	1 guava (2.8 oz.)	1	1	4	4	283	1	2	0	1	49	102	Extremely high in vitamin C.
Haddock, fried	3 oz.	23	0	2	3	0	3	5	9	45	135	2	Rich in minerals from the ocean.
Halibut, broiled	1 piece (3 oz.)	32	7	2	3	0	2	7	12	60	155	2	Contains vit. D which is scarce in foods grown in soil.
Ham: Smoked	3 oz.	26	0	24	8	0	4	12	81	216	290	3	
Sliced luncheon meat	1 oz.	9	0	2	4	0	0	8	22	58	85	3	High in fat calories.
Hamburger: Broiled (ground lean)	3 oz.	33	1	5	11	0	1	30	45	90	185	4	
Broiled (market ground)	3 oz.	30	0	4	7	0	1	27	72	153	245	2	62% of the calories are from fat.
Hamburger with bun	One (meat 1.5 oz., bun 1.8 oz.)	21	0	10	7	0	6	27	44	77	254	3	
Hard candy	1 oz.	0	0	0	0	0	0	0	0	0	110	0	Empty calories.
Heart, beef, braised (fat trimmed)	3 oz.	37	1	14	58	4	2	59	18	45	160	14	High in protein, B complex vitamins, and iron.
Herring, smoked, kippered	3 oz.	27	0	0	13	0	7	12	18	99	180	3	Low in saturated fat.

HEALTH-BUILDING VALUES OF FOODS

FOOD	AMOUNT	PROTEIN	Vitamin A	Vitamin B₁	Vitamin B₂	Vitamin C	Calcium	Iron	Saturated Fat Calories	Total Fat Calories (Both saturated and unsaturated)	TOTAL CALORIES (From protein, fat, and carbohydrate)	V-M INDEX	REMARKS (The Vitamin-Mineral Index is shown at left. The higher the Index number, the more vitamins and minerals per calorie of food.)
Highball	1 glass (4.3 oz.)	0	0	0	0	0	0	0	0	0	170	0	
Hominy	1/2 cup (0.7 oz.)	2	0	3	2	0	0	4	0	1	60	3	
Honey	1 tablespoon (0.7 oz.)	0	1	0	1	1	3	6	0	0	60	1	Good source of vitamin C.
Honeydew melon	1 medium slice (5.3 oz.)	1	1	4	2	45	3	8	0	0	49	21	
Hot dog without bun	1 hot dog (1.8 oz.)	9	0	5	6	0	0	8	54	126	155	2	Note high amount of fat.
Hot dog including bun	One (dog 1.8 oz., bun 1.7 oz.)	16	0	7	8	0	3	12	63	144	315	2	
Ice cream, plain	1 small scoop (2.2 oz.)	3	6	2	7	1	10	1	36	72	130	3	
Ice cream cone, vanilla	1 sm. scoop with cone (2.4 oz.)	3	6	2	7	1	10	1	37	75	146	3	
Ice milk	1 small scoop (2.2 oz.)	6	3	2	10	1	16	1	23	39	124	4	Lower in fat calories.
Jams, marmalades, preserves	1 tablespoon (0.7 oz.)	0	0	0	1	1	1	1	0	0	55	1	
Jellies	1 tablespoon (0.7 oz.)	0	0	0	0	1	0	0	0	0	50	1	
Jello-type dessert	1/2 cup (4.2 oz.)	3	0	0	0	0	0	0	0	0	78	0	
Jello-type dessert with fruit	1/2 cup (4.2 oz.)	2	3	2	1	5	1	4	0	1	85	3	
Kale, cooked	1/2 cup (1.9 oz.)	3	92	2	7	37	16	12	0	4	22	121	Excellent in vitamins A & C - low in calories.
Kidney beans, cooked	1/2 cup (4.5 oz.)	11	4	4	4	0	5	23	0	0	115	5	
Kidneys, beef, cooked	3 oz.	35	38	30	230	28	2	128	60	119	230	33	Rich in protein, iron, and B complex vitamins.
Kohlrabi, raw	1/2 cup (2.4 oz.)	2	0	2	2	56	4	4	0	0	20	57	Fine source of vit. C - good for modern low calorie meals.
Lamb cooked: Chop, broiled	1 chop (4 oz.)	36	0	9	14	0	1	31	162	297	405	2	
Chop, broiled (fat trimmed)	1 chop (2.6 oz.)	30	0	7	11	0	1	25	27	54	140	5	Trimming helps you lower your fat total.
Leg of lamb	3 oz.	31	0	8	13	0	1	28	81	144	235	4	
Leg of lamb (fat trimmed)	3 oz.	34	0	9	14	0	1	31	32	54	156	6	Trimming outside fat reduces saturated fat calories.
Liver, fried	1 piece (3 oz.)	30	1046	21	184	37	1	126	40	71	177	133	Extremely high in vitamin A.
Shoulder roast	3 oz.	26	0	7	11	0	1	24	117	207	285	3	
Shoulder roast (fat trimmed)	3 oz.	32	0	8	13	0	1	29	35	71	173	5	Trimming fat helps fight high cholesterol level.
Lard	1 tablespoon (1/2 oz.)	0	0	0	0	0	0	0	45	126	126	0	
Layer cake with icing	2" sector of 10" diam. cake (3.5 oz.)	7	2	1	4	1	15	4	18	54	320	1	
Lemons	1 medium (3.7 oz.)	1	0	2	1	51	2	4	0	2	20	50	High in vitamin C.
Lemon juice, fresh	1 tablespoon (1/2 oz.)	0	0	0	0	9	0	0	0	1	5	30	
Lemonade, made from frozen concentrate, sweetened	1 cup ready to drink (8 fl. oz.)	0	0	1	1	23	0	1	0	2	110	4	
Lemon meringue pie	4" sector of 9" diam. pie (4.2 oz.)	6	4	2	6	1	3	6	36	108	300	1	
Lettuce, head type	1/4 head (4 oz.)	2	12	3	5	12	3	6	0	2	17	39	Excellent for vitamins, minerals, and roughage.
Lettuce leaves, head type	2 large or 4 small (1.8 oz.)	1	5	1	5	5	3	2	0	2	7	39	
Lima beans: Baby, cooked	1/2 cup (2.8 oz.)	6	5	7	4	16	3	14	0	4	75	11	
Dried, cooked	1/2 cup (3.4 oz.)	11	0	8	3	0	4	28	0	4	130	6	
Limburger cheese	1 piece (1 oz.)	9	7	1	8	0	21	2	39	71	97	7	
Limes	1 medium 2" diam. (2.4 oz.)	1	0	1	0	19	3	3	0	1	19	23	Makes a low calorie drink rich in vitamin C.

HEALTH-BUILDING VALUES OF FOODS

FOOD	AMOUNT	PROTEIN	Vitamin A	Vitamin B₁	Vitamin B₂	Vitamin C	Calcium	Iron	Saturated Fat Calories	Total Fat Calories (Both saturated and unsaturated)	TOTAL CALORIES (From protein, fat, and carbohydrate)	V-M INDEX	REMARKS
					% OF DAILY ALLOWANCE								(The Vitamin-Mineral Index is shown at left. The higher the Index number, the more vitamins and minerals per calorie of food.)
Lime juice: Fresh	1 tablespoon (1.4 oz.)	0	0	0	0	7	0	0	0	0	4	29	
Canned	1 tablespoon (1.4 oz.)	0	0	0	0	4	0	0	0	0	4	17	
Limeade, made from frozen concentrate, sweetened	1 cup ready to drink (8 fl. oz.)	0	0	1	0	8	0	2	2	2	105	2	
Liquor and alcoholic beverages: Ale	1 can (12 fl. oz.)	2	0	0	6	0	6	3	0	0	148	2	
Beer	1 can (12 fl. oz.)	2	0	0	5	0	2	0	0	3	171	1	
Brandy, 86 proof	1 jigger (1-1/2 oz.)	0	0	0	0	0	0	0	0	0	108	0	Most liquor is loaded with empty calories.
Champagne	3 oz. glass	0	0	0	0	0	0	0	0	0	75	0	
Cordials and liqueurs, 80 proof	1 jigger (1-1/2 oz.)	0	0	0	0	0	1	1	0	0	146	0	
Daiquiri cocktail	1 cocktail	0	0	1	0	11	1	1	0	0	124	2	
Gin, 94 proof	1 jigger (1-1/2 oz.)	0	0	0	0	0	0	0	0	0	119	3	
Highball	1 glass	0	0	0	0	0	0	0	0	0	170	0	
Manhattan cocktail	1 cocktail	0	1	2	0	0	0	0	0	0	167	0	
Martini cocktail	1 cocktail	0	0	0	0	0	1	1	0	0	143	0	
Old fashioned cocktail	1 glass	0	0	0	0	0	1	0	0	0	183	0	
Rum, 86 proof	1 jigger (1-1/2 oz.)	0	0	0	0	0	0	0	0	0	108	0	This "demon" lacks vitamins and minerals.
Tom Collins cocktail	1 cocktail	0	0	2	0	28	1	0	0	0	182	3	
Vermouth	3 oz. glass	0	0	0	0	0	0	0	0	0	150	0	
Vodka, 100 proof	1 jigger (1-1/2 oz.)	0	0	0	0	0	0	0	0	0	126	0	Guaranteed to contain no vitamins or minerals.
Whiskey, 86 proof	1 jigger (1-1/2 oz.)	0	0	0	0	0	0	1	0	0	108	0	
Whiskey, 100 proof	1 jigger (1-1/2 oz.)	0	0	0	0	0	0	0	0	0	126	0	
Wine, kosher	4 oz. glass	0	0	0	0	0	0	0	0	0	127	0	
Wine, dry sherry	3 oz. glass	0	0	0	0	0	0	0	0	0	124	0	
Liver: Beef, fried	1 piece (3 oz.)	28	910	14	188	36	1	66	27	54	180	112	Outstanding in protein, vitamins, and minerals.
Calf liver, fried	1 piece (3 oz.)	28	466	11	175	40	1	106	45	91	184	72	Liver is one of the most nutritious foods you can eat.
Chicken liver, fried	3 chicken livers (3 oz.)	32	667	11	139	23	2	74	24	74	184	83	Liver contains nutrients not yet identified.
Lamb liver, fried	1 piece (3 oz.)	30	1046	21	184	37	1	126	40	71	177	133	Extremely high in vitamin A.
Pork liver, fried	1 piece (3 oz.)	29	294	21	167	25	1	181	30	89	174	66	Liver is an outstanding source of B complex vitamins and vitamin A.
Liver sausage or liverwurst	1 oz.	7	33	3	18	0	0	16	25	53	75	16	The most nutritious of the luncheon meats.
Lobster, canned	3 oz.	22	0	2	3	0	7	7	2	10	78	4	High quality protein with little fat.
Loganberries, fresh	1/2 cup (2.5 oz.)	1	3	1	3	23	3	7	0	4	45	15	
Macaroni, cooked	1/2 cup (2.5 oz.)	4	0	6	3	0	3	6	0	4	78	3	
Macaroni and cheese, baked	1/2 cup (3.9 oz.)	13	10	7	13	0	25	10	63	112	238	5	
Mackerel, broiled	3 oz.	27	9	8	13	0	1	10	23	117	200	5	
Malted milk	1 cup (8 fl. oz.)	19	13	11	31	3	46	8	63	108	280	7	
Mango, fresh	1 medium (7.1 oz.)	1	168	5	4	73	2	3	0	3	87	49	Excellent in vitamins A and C

228

HEALTH-BUILDING VALUES OF FOODS

FOOD	AMOUNT	% OF DAILY ALLOWANCE							Saturated Fat Calories	Total Fat Calories (Both saturated and unsaturated)	TOTAL CALORIES (From protein, fat, and carbohydrate)	V-M INDEX	REMARKS (The Vitamin-Mineral Index is shown at left. The higher the Index number, the more vitamins and minerals per calorie of food.)
		PROTEIN	Vitamin A	Vitamin B_1	Vitamin B_2	Vitamin C	Calcium	Iron					
Manhattan cocktail	1 cocktail	0	0	0	0	0	0	0	0	0	167	0	
Margarine	1 pat (1/4 oz.)	0	5	0	0	0	0	0	14	50	50	2	Has less saturated fat than butter.
Margarine (made especially low in saturated fat)	1 tablespoon (1/2 oz.)	0	9	0	0	0	0	0	27	100	100	2	Has less saturated fat than regular margarine.
Marmalade	1 tablespoon (1/2 oz.)	0	0	0	0	1	0	1	0	0	55	2	
Marshmallow	1 oz.	1	0	0	0	0	0	1	0	0	90	1	Dentists deplore these relatively empty calories.
Martini	1 cocktail	1	0	0	0	0	0	1	0	0	143	0	
Mayonnaise	1 tablespoon (1/2 oz.)	0	1	0	0	0	0	1	18	108	110	0	Low in saturated fat – high in desirable linoleic fat.
Milk: Whole milk	1 cup (8 fl. oz.)	12	8	6	23	4	36	2	47	86	166	8	The best source of calcium.
	1 quart (32 fl. oz.)	49	31	22	93	17	144	7	189	343	666	8	
Skim milk	1 cup (8 fl. oz.)	12	0	6	24	4	38	1	2	2	87	14	Excellent in protein and calcium with little saturated fat.
	1 quart (32 fl. oz.)	49	1	22	97	17	151	7	5	9	350	14	
Milk made from nonfat skim milk power	1 cup ready to drink (8 fl. oz.)	12	0	6	24	4	38	2	1	2	87	14	Use this generously and avoid saturated butter fat.
	1 quart ready to drink (32 fl. oz.)	49	1	22	97	17	144	7	5	9	348	14	
Buttermilk	1 cup (8 fl. oz.)	11	1	6	23	4	34	4	2	9	87	14	Helps you avoid saturated fat.
Chocolate milk	1 cup (8 fl. oz.)	11	2	6	15	3	39	2	54	90	190	6	
Evaporated milk, undiluted	1 cup (8 fl. oz.)	26	16	6	47	4	79	3	99	180	345	7	
Condensed milk, sweetened	1 tablespoon (0.7 oz.)	2	1	1	4	0	6	0	14	14	62	3	
Dry whole milk powder	1 cup of powder (3.6 oz.)	39	23	19	83	8	121	5	135	252	515	5	For added nutrition, blend in mashed potatoes, soups, stews.
Dry nonfat skim milk powder	1 tablespoon of powder (0.2 oz.)	3	1	1	5	1	8	0	0	0	18	14	
	1 cup of powder (2.8 oz.)	41	1	18	80	1	130	5	0	9	290	14	
Malted milk	1 cup (8 fl. oz.)	19	13	11	31	3	46	8	63	108	280	7	
Goat's milk	1 cup (8 fl. oz.)	11	8	6	15	3	39	2	54	90	165	7	
Soybean milk (without enrichment)	1 cup (8 fl. oz.)	11	0	12	6	1	6	16	18	31	76	9	May be used by those allergic to milk – low in calcium.
Mince pie	4" sector of 9" diam. pie (4.8 oz.)	4	0	1	1	1	3	9	18	81	340	5	
Molasses: Light cane	1 tablespoon (0.7 oz.)	0	0	1	1	0	4	9	0	0	50	15	
Blackstrap	1 tablespoon (0.7 oz.)	0	0	1	2	0	14	23	0	0	45	15	This food is an excellent natural laxative.
Muffins: Made w/ enriched white flour	1 muffin 2-3/4" diam. (1.7 oz.)	6	1	5	6	0	9	7	9	45	135	3	
Corn muffins w/enriched meal	1 muffin (1.7 oz.)	6	3	6	8	0	10	9	18	45	155	4	
Mung bean sprouts, fresh	1/2 cup (1.6 oz.)	2	2	2	2	9	2	4	0	0	10	32	A crunchy addition to salads – delicious when steamed.
Mushrooms, canned	1/4 cup (2.2 oz.)	1	0	1	8	1	1	4	0	6	8	31	Adds flavor and variety to modern low calorie meals.
Mushroom cream soup	1 cup (8 fl. oz.)	10	4	3	11	0	27	5	63	108	200	4	
Muskmelons	1/2 melon (13.6 oz.)	1	132	6	4	84	4	8	0	2	40	99	Fine for vitamins A and C – low in calories.

HEALTH-BUILDING VALUES OF FOODS

FOOD	AMOUNT	PROTEIN	Vitamin A	Vitamin B₁	Vitamin B₂	Vitamin C	Calcium	Iron	Saturated Fat Calories	Total Fat Calories (Both saturated and unsaturated)	TOTAL CALORIES (From protein, fat, and carbohydrate)	V-M INDEX	REMARKS (The Vitamin-Mineral Index is shown at left. The higher the Index number, the more vitamins and minerals per calorie of food.)
Mustard greens, cooked	1/2 cup (2.5 oz.)	2	101	2	7	42	19	20	0	1	15	212	High in vitamins A, C, calcium & iron - very low in calories.
Navy beans, cooked	1/2 cup (4.5 oz.)	11	0	4	4	0	5	23	0	4	115	5	
Noodles: Egg noodles, cooked, enriched	1/2 cup (2.8 oz.)	5	1	7	4	0	1	7	4	9	100	3	
Egg noodles, cooked, unenriched	1/2 cup (2.8 oz.)	5	1	1	1	0	1	5	4	9	100	2	
Noodle soup	1 cup (8 fl. oz.)	9	1	1	3	0	10	2	9	36	115	2	
Nuts: Almonds	14 almonds (1/2 oz.)	4	0	2	7	0	4	7	5	69	85	4	Has complete protein and desirable unsaturated fat.
Brazil nuts	1 tbsp. broken pieces (0.3 oz.)	2	0	5	0	0	2	3	10	52	57	3	Rich in linoleic fat.
Cashew, roasted	1 tablespoon (0.3 oz.)	2	0	2	2	0	0	3	6	37	48	2	
Peanuts	1 oz.	11	1	6	2	0	2	6	29	126	165	2	A nutritious snack to use in place of candy.
Pecans	1 tbsp. chopped nuts (0.3 oz.)	1	0	4	1	0	1	2	2	45	50	3	Has valuable unsaturated fat.
Black walnuts	1 tbsp. chopped nuts (0.3 oz.)	2	0	1	0	0	1	5	2	42	49	2	High in linoleic fat.
English walnuts	1 tbsp. chopped nuts (0.3 oz.)	1	0	2	0	0	0	2	2	45	50	2	An excellent source of desirable linoleic fat.
Oat cereal mixture, enriched	1 oz.	6	0	14	2	0	6	12	2	18	115	5	
Oatmeal or rolled oats	1/2 cup (4.2 oz.)	4	0	7	1	0	1	8	2	14	75	4	
Oil: Corn oil such as Mazola	1 tablespoon (1/2 oz.)	0	0	0	0	0	0	0	18	125	125	0	Rich in desirable unsaturated linoleic fat.
Cottonseed oil such as Wesson	1 tablespoon (1/2 oz.)	0	0	0	0	0	0	0	27	125	125	0	Rich in desirable unsaturated linoleic fat.
Olive oil	1 tablespoon (1/2 oz.)	0	0	0	0	0	0	0	18	125	125	0	Rich in unsaturated fat though low in linoleic fat.
Soybean oil	1 tablespoon (1/2 oz.)	0	0	0	0	0	0	0	18	125	125	0	High in helpful linoleic fat.
Okra, cooked	8 medium pods (3 oz.)	3	13	3	3	23	9	6	0	2	30	32	Rich in vitamins and minerals.
Old fashioned cocktail	1 glass	0	0	0	0	0	0	0	0	0	183	0	
Olives: Green	6 extra lg. or 3-1/2 jumbo (1.2 oz.)	1	2	0	0	0	3	4	3	29	32	5	
Ripe or black	6 extra lg. or 3-1/2 jumbo (1.2 oz.)	1	0	0	0	0	3	4	4	40	42	3	
Olive oil	1 tablespoon (1/2 oz.)	0	0	0	0	0	0	0	18	125	125	0	Rich in unsaturated fat though low in linoleic fat.
Onion	1 onion 2-1/2" diam. (3.9 oz.)	3	1	2	2	13	4	6	0	0	50	9	
Spring onions	2 stalks (0.6 oz.)	0	0	0	0	5	3	1	0	1	8	19	
Orange, fresh	One 3" diam. orange (7.4 oz.)	1	6	8	2	88	8	3	0	2	70	27	Rich in vitamin C - has desirable pectin and roughage when pulp is eaten.
Orange Juice: Fresh	1/2 cup (4 fl. oz.)	1	5	7	2	81	2	4	0	4	60	28	Wonderful for vitamin C.
Canned	1/2 cup (4 fl. oz.)	1	5	5	1	67	2	5	0	1	60	24	
Juice made from frozen concentrate	1/2 cup ready to drink (4 fl. oz.)	1	5	7	2	75	1	2	0	1	55	27	Use orange juice generously to build your vit. C total.
Juice made from powder	1/2 cup ready to drink (4 fl. oz.)	1	5	6	2	72	2	2	0	1	58	26	
Orange and grapefruit juice made from frozen concentrate	1/2 cup ready to drink (4 fl. oz.)	1	3	5	1	68	1	1	0	1	55	24	
Oysters, raw without shell	1/2 cup, about 8 med. (4.2 oz.)	14	7	9	11	0	14	66	4	18	80	22	Complete protein with low fat content - rich in iron.
Oyster stew, with milk	1 cup with 3 to 4 oysters (8 fl. oz.)	16	13	8	22	0	34	33	22	108	200	9	
Oyster crackers	10 crackers (0.4 oz.)	1	0	1	0	0	0	1	4	9	45	1	

HEALTH-BUILDING VALUES OF FOODS

FOOD	AMOUNT	PROTEIN	Vitamin A	Vitamin B₁	Vitamin B₂	Vitamin C	Calcium	Iron	Saturated Fat Calories	Total Fat Calories (Both saturated and unsaturated)	TOTAL CALORIES (From protein, fat, and carbohydrate)	V-M INDEX	REMARKS (The Vitamin-Mineral Index is shown at left. The higher the Index number, the more vitamins and minerals per calorie of food.)
Pancakes made with enriched flour	One 4" diam. (1 oz.)	3	1	3	3	0	4	3	2	18	60	4	
Made from buckwheat pancake mix	1 pancake (1 oz.)	3	1	2	2	0	8	3	9	18	45	6	Contains an enzyme that aids digestion.
Papaya	1/2 cup (3.2 oz.)	1	32	1	2	68	2	2	1	1	35	51	
Parmesan cheese	1 piece (1 oz.)	15	6	1	12	0	41	1	37	67	112	9	High in calcium.
Parsley, chopped	1 tablespoon (0.1 oz.)	0	6	0	1	9	1	2	0	0	1	317	Has extraordinary vitamins & minerals per calorie.
Parsnips, cooked	1/2 cup (2.7 oz.)	1	1	3	4	13	6	6	0	4	48	11	
Peaches: Fresh	1 peach 2" diam. (4 oz.)	1	26	1	3	9	1	6	0	2	35	21	Use fruit to replace gooey desserts.
Fresh, sliced	1/2 cup (3 oz.)	1	22	1	3	8	1	4	0	1	33	19	A good source of vitamin A.
Canned with water	1/2 cup (4.3 oz.)	1	11	1	2	5	1	4	0	1	38	11	
Canned with syrup	1/2 cup (4.5 oz.)	1	11	1	2	5	1	4	0	1	100	4	Added sugar ups the calories.
Dried and cooked, unsweetened	2 halves w/2 tbsps. syrup (4.1 oz.)	0	10	1	2	4	1	4	0	2	90	4	
Peach nectar	1/2 cup (4.8 oz.)	2	33	0	4	4	2	26	0	4	110	10	
Peanuts	1/2 cup (4 fl. oz.)	11	0	6	2	1	2	6	29	126	165	5	A nutritious snack to use in place of candy.
Peanut brittle	1 oz.	3	0	2	1	0	2	4		40	125	2	
Peanut butter	1 tablespoon (0.6 oz.)	6	0	1	1	0	2	4	18	72	90	1	More nutritious than jelly or jam.
Pears: Fresh	1 pear (6.4 oz.)	1	1	2	4	9	2	5	1	9	100	4	An excellent dessert or between-meal snack.
Canned with syrup	2 halves w/2 tbsps. syrup (4.1 oz.)	0	1	0	1	3	1	1	0	1	90	1	
Pear nectar	1/2 cup (4 fl. oz.)	1	0	0	1	1	1	1	0	1	65	1	
Peas, green: Fresh, cooked	1/2 cup (2.8 oz.)	6	12	12	6	16	2	15	0	4	55	19	
Canned	1/2 cup (4.4 oz.)	6	14	9	4	14	4	22	0	4	85	13	
Dry split peas, cooked	1/2 cup (4.4 oz.)	14	4	11	6	0	2	21	0	4	145	5	
Peas, blackeyed, cooked	1/2 cup (4.4 oz.)	9	9	13	3	0	3	16	0	4	95	6	
Pea soup	1 cup (8 fl. oz.)	9	9	11	4	7	4	15	9	18	140	6	
Pecans	1 tablespoon chopped nuts (0.3 oz.)	1	0	4	1	0	1	2	2	45	50	3	Has valuable unsaturated fat.
Peppers: Green, without seeds, raw	1 medium pepper (2.2 oz.)	1	5	3	3	105	1	4	0	2	15	134	Very high in vitamin C.
Sweet, red pod without seeds, raw	1 medium pepper (2.1 oz.)	1	53	3	3	163	1	4	0	2	20	189	Excellent for vitamin C - rich in vitamin A.
Canned pimientos	1 medium pimiento (1.3 oz.)	0	17	1	1	48	0	6	0	2	10	122	High in vitamin C.
Powder, red hot chili powder	1 teaspoon (0.2 oz.)	1	77	1	4	1	1	4	0	3	17	86	
Perch, ocean perch breaded and fried	3 oz.	23	1	6	6	0	2	13	20	99	195	2	Fish are ideal for modern diets.
Persimmons, fresh	1 persimmon (4.4 oz.)	1	55	2	1	15	1	4	0	2	75	17	Rich in vitamin A.
Pickles: Dill	1 pickle 4" long (4.8 oz.)	0	8	0	5	11	4	16	0	2	15	49	
Sweet	1 pickle 2-3/4" long (0.7 oz.)	0	0	0	1	1	0	3	0	2	20	3	
Cucumber bread & butter pickles	6 slices (1.5 oz.)	1	2	1	1	5	2	4	0	1	29	11	
Piecrust: Lower crust	1 piecrust 9" diam. (4.8 oz.)	14	0	18	13	0	4	27	72	324	655	2	
Double crust	1 piecrust 9" diam. (9.5 oz.)	29	0	36	26	0	4	54	153	657	1315	2	
Pies: Apple	4" sector of 9" diam. pie (4.8 oz.)	4	4	2	1	1	1	5	36	117	330	1	Most pies are high in calories.

231

HEALTH-BUILDING VALUES OF FOODS

FOOD	AMOUNT	PROTEIN	Vitamin A	Vitamin B₁	Vitamin B₂	Vitamin C	Calcium	Iron	Saturated Fat Calories	Total Fat Calories (Both saturated and unsaturated)	TOTAL CALORIES (From protein, fat, and carbohydrate)	V-M INDEX	REMARKS (The Vitamin-Mineral Index is shown at left. The higher the Index number, the more vitamins and minerals per calorie of food.)
Pies: Cherry	4" sector of 9" diam. pie (4.8 oz.)	4	10	2	1	3	1	5	36	117	340	1	
Custard	4" sector of 9" diam. pie (4.6 oz.)	10	6	4	12	0	20	16	36	99	265	4	
Lemon meringue	4" sector of 9" diam. pie (4.2 oz.)	6	4	2	6	1	3	6	36	108	300	1	
Mince	4" sector of 9" diam. pie (4.8 oz.)	4	0	6	3	1	3	30	18	81	340	2	
Pumpkin	4" sector of 9" diam. pie (4.6 oz.)	7	50	2	8	0	9	10	45	108	265	5	High in vitamin A.
Pimientos, canned	1 medium pimiento (1.3 oz.)	0	17	1	1	48	0	6	0	2	10	122	High in vitamin C.
Pineapple: Fresh, diced	1/2 cup (2.5 oz.)	1	1	4	1	22	1	8	0	1	38	14	
Crushed with syrup	1/2 cup (4.6 oz.)	1	2	6	1	15	5	4	0	1	102	6	
Rings, with syrup	2 small or 1 large ring (4.3 oz.)	0	2	6	1	15	4	7	0	2	95	6	
Pineapple juice	1/2 cup (4 fl. oz.)	1	2	4	1	15	3	6	0	1	60	8	
Pizza, cheese	5-1/2" sector of 14" pie (2.6 oz.)	11	11	2	5	11	20	7	27	54	180	5	
Plums: Fresh	1 medium plum (2.1 oz.)	0	4	2	1	4	1	2	0	2	30	8	
Canned with syrup	3 plums, 2 tbsps. juice (4.3 oz.)	0	6	2	2	1	1	13	0	2	90	2	
Popcorn, popped	1 cup (1/2 oz.)	3	0	3	1	0	0	4	1	9	55	5	
Pork, cooked: Chop	1 chop (3-1/2 oz.)	23	0	39	10	0	1	22	72	189	260	5	
Chop (fat trimmed)	1 chop (1.7 oz.)	21	0	34	9	0	1	19	27	63	130	8	Calories cut in half when fat trimmed – other nutrients largely unchanged.
Ham, smoked	3 oz.	26	0	24	8	0	1	22	81	216	290	3	
Liver, fried	1 piece (3 oz.)	29	294	21	167	25	1	181	30	89	174	66	Liver is an outstanding source of B complex vitamins and vitamin A.
Roast	3 oz.	30	0	49	12	0	1	27	81	216	310	5	By trimming the fat you help hold down your cholesterol.
Roast (fat trimmed)	3 oz.	36	0	57	14	0	1	27	45	112	219	8	
Sausage	2 oz.	13	0	7	8	0	1	13	45	130	170	3	
Various cuts, simmered	3 oz.	29	0	29	12	0	1	25	81	234	320	3	
Various cuts, simmered (fat trimmed)	3 oz.	35	0	35	14	0	1	31	24	73	182	7	
Pork and beans with sauce	1/2 cup (4.6 oz.)	11	1	4	3	3	11	22	14	32	165	4	
Pot roast, cooked: Beef	3 oz.	33	1	2	10	0	1	29	72	144	245	5	
Beef (fat trimmed)	3 oz.	37	0	3	11	0	1	32	20	53	165	5	Trimming off fat may help your arteries.
Potatoes: Baked, peeled after baking	1 potato (3.5 oz.)	4	0	6	2	27	1	7	0	2	90	8	
Boiled, peeled after boiling	1 potato (4.8 oz.)	4	0	8	3	29	1	8	0	2	105	8	
French fried	10 pieces 2" long, 1/2" sq. (2 oz.)	3	0	4	2	11	1	7	18	63	155	3	
Mashed, milk added	1/2 cup (3.4 oz.)	3	1	5	3	11	3	5	1	4	72	6	
Mashed, milk and butter added	1/2 cup (3.4 oz.)	3	5	5	3	11	3	5	32	54	115	5	
Potato chips	10 chips 2" diam. (0.7 oz.)	1	0	2	1	3	1	4	18	63	110	2	
Potpie, beef, baked	1 pie 4-1/2" diam. (8 oz.)	26	57	4	8	0	2	25	90	252	460	3	
Pound cake	2-3/4"x3"x5/8" (1.1 oz.)	3	2	2	3	0	2	5	18	63	130	2	
Preserves	1 tablespoon (0.7 oz.)	0	0	0	0	1	0	1	0	2	55	1	

HEALTH-BUILDING VALUES OF FOODS

FOOD	AMOUNT	PROTEIN	Vitamin A	Vitamin B₁	Vitamin B₂	Vitamin C	Calcium	Iron	Saturated Fat Calories	Total Fat Calories (Both saturated and unsaturated)	TOTAL CALORIES (From protein, fat, and carbohydrate)	V-M INDEX	REMARKS (The Vitamin-Mineral Index is shown at left. The higher the Index number, the more vitamins and minerals per calorie of food.)
Pretzels	5 small sticks (0.2 oz.)	0	0	0	0	0	0	0	0	2	20	0	
Prunes: Cooked, unsweetened	1/2 cup (4.8 oz.)	2	18	0	5	2	4	22	0	4	152	6	
Dried	4 medium prunes (1.1 oz.)	1	9	1	3	1	2	10	0	2	70	6	A natural laxative.
Prune juice, canned	1/2 cup (4 fl. oz.)	1	0	0	1	3	2	49	0	1	85	11	
Prune whip dessert	1/2 cup (2.4 oz.)	3	12	2	4	1	2	12	0	2	100	6	
Pudding, cornstarch (Blanc mange)	1/2 cup (4.4 oz.)	6	4	2	11	1	18	0	27	45	138	4	
Pumpernickel bread, dark	1 slice (0.8 oz.)	3	0	3	2	0	2	6	1	2	56	4	High in vitamin A.
Pumpkin, canned	1/2 cup (4 oz.)	1	78	1	4	0	3	8	1	4	38	41	High in vitamin A.
Pumpkin pie	4" sector of 9" diam. pie (4.6 oz.)	7	50	2	8	0	9	10	45	108	265	5	High in vitamin A.
Radishes, tops removed	4 small (1.4 oz.)	0	0	1	1	13	2	4	0	2	10	35	Raw foods like this are negligible in calories and very filling.
Raisin Bran cereal	1 cup (1.8 oz.)	6	0	12	5	0	4	24	1	8	149	5	
Raisin bread	1 slice (0.8 oz.)	3	0	1	1	0	2	3	1	9	60	2	
Raisins	1 tablespoon (0.4 oz.)	0	0	1	0	0	1	4	0	0	29	3	
Raspberries: Red fresh	1/2 cup (2.2 oz.)	1	2	1	2	21	2	6	0	4	35	16	
Black fresh	1/2 cup (2.4 oz.)	1	0	1	2	21	3	6	1	14	50	11	
Rhubarb, cooked with sugar	1/2 cup (4.8 oz.)	1	1	1	0	11	6	3	0	1	192	2	83% of the calories are fat calories.
Rib roast, cooked: Beef	3 oz.	23	1	2	7	0	1	21	153	324	390	1	Modern folks trim the fat off for improved nutrition.
Beef (fat trimmed)	3 oz.	33	0	4	10	0	1	30	45	105	200	4	
Rice: White rice, cooked	1/2 cup (3 oz.)	3	0	1	0	0	1	2	0	1	100	1	
Converted white rice, cooked	1/2 cup (3.1 oz.)	3	0	3	1	0	1	2	0	1	102	1	
Brown rice, cooked	1/2 cup (4.2 oz.)	3	0	8	1	0	1	6	0	4	101	2	
Wild rice, cooked	1/2 cup (2.4 oz.)	7	0	8	13	0	1	8	0	2	135	3	
Rice bran	1 oz.	6	0	40	4	0	3	58	6	36	80	22	One of the best sources of B complex vitamins.
Rice cereals: Puffed rice	1 cup (1/2 oz.)	1	0	4	1	0	0	2	0	2	55	2	
Rice flakes	1 cup (1.1 oz.)	3	0	7	1	0	1	5	0	1	115	2	
Rice polish (a powder)	1 oz.	4	0	32	3	0	2	46	0	36	70	20	This powder (made when rice is polished) is rich in B vits.
Rice soup	1 cup (8 fl. oz.)	9	1	1	3	0	10	2	6	36	115	2	
Roasts cooked: Beef, fatty cut such as rib	3 oz.	23	1	4	7	0	1	21	153	324	390	1	83% of the calories are fat calories.
Beef, fatty cut (outside fat trimmed)	3 oz.	33	1	4	10	0	1	30	45	105	220	4	Modern folks trim the fat off for improved nutrition.
Beef, lean cut such as round	3 oz.	33	1	4	10	0	1	30	63	126	220	3	
Beef, lean cut (outside fat trimmed)	3 oz.	36	0	4	11	0	1	32	22	43	156	5	Reduce your saturated fat calories by trimming.
Beef, veal roast	3 oz.	33	0	7	14	0	1	29	63	126	305	3	
Lamb shoulder roast	3 oz.	26	0	7	11	0	1	24	117	207	285	3	
Lamb shoulder roast (outside fat trimmed)	3 oz.	32	0	8	13	1	1	29	35	71	173	5	Trimming fat helps fight high cholesterol level.

HEALTH-BUILDING VALUES OF FOODS

FOOD	AMOUNT	PROTEIN	Vitamin A	Vitamin B₁	Vitamin B₂	Vitamin C	Calcium	Iron	Saturated Fat Calories	Total Fat Calories (Both saturated and unsaturated)	TOTAL CALORIES (From protein, fat, and carbohydrate)	V-M INDEX	REMARKS (The Vitamin-Mineral Index is shown at left. The higher the Index number, the more vitamins and minerals per calorie of food.)
Roasts cooked: Pork roast	3 oz.	30	0	49	12	0	1	27	81	216	310	5	
Pork roast (outside fat trimmed)	3 oz.	36	0	57	14	0	1	32	45	112	219	8	By trimming the fat you help hold down your cholesterol.
Rolls: Hard round roll	1 roll (1.8 oz.)	7	0	2	3	0	3	4	9	18	160	1	
Soft roll, enriched flour	1 roll (1.3 oz.)	4	0	7	4	0	4	3	9	18	115	3	
Sweet roll	1 roll (1.5 oz.)	6	1	2	3	0	5	3	9	36	135	2	
Roquefort cheese	1 oz.	9	7	1	9	0	15	2	45	81	105	5	High in saturated fat.
Roquefort salad dressing	1 tablespoon (0.6 oz.)	1	1	0	1	0	1	0	18	86	90	1	Contains valuable linoleic fat.
Round steak: Beef, broiled	3 oz.	34	0	4	11	0	1	30	54	117	220	3	Leaner meats contain more protein.
Round steak, broiled (fat trimmed)	3 oz.	39	0	4	11	0	1	32	22	44	160	5	Note drop in saturated fat calories.
Rum, 86 proof	1 jigger (1-1/2 oz.)	0	0	0	0	0	0	0	0	0	108	0	This "demon" lacks vitamins and minerals.
Rutabaga, cooked	1/2 cup (2.7 oz.)	1	5	2	3	22	5	3	0	1	25	27	
Rye bread	1 slice (0.8 oz.)	3	0	2	1	0	2	4	0	2	55	3	
Rye wafers such as Ry-Krisp	2 wafers about 2"x3" (1/2 oz.)	3	0	2	2	0	1	6	0	2	42	4	
Salad dressing: Blue Cheese or Roquefort	1 tablespoon (0.6 oz.)	1	1	0	1	0	1	0	18	86	90	4	Contains valuable linoleic fat.
French dressing	1 tablespoon (1/2 oz.)	0	1	0	0	0	1	1	18	48	60	0	Good source of desirable linoleic fat.
Home cooked, boiled	1 tablespoon (0.6 oz.)	1	2	1	2	0	2	1	9	18	30	4	Low in saturated fat - high in desirable linoleic fat.
Mayonnaise	1 tablespoon (1/2 oz.)	0	1	0	0	0	0	1	18	108	110	0	Good source of desirable linoleic fat.
Mayonnaise-type salad dressing	1 tablespoon (1/2 oz.)	0	1	0	0	0	0	1	9	54	60	1	High in linoleic fat.
Thousand Island	1 tablespoon (1/2 oz.)	0	1	0	0	3	0	1	9	72	75		Contains the elusive vitamin D.
Salmon, canned	3 oz.	24	1	2	9	0	20	7	9	45	120	5	
Saltines	2 crackers 2" square (0.3 oz.)	1	0	0	0	0	0	1	9	9	35	2	Crackers are high in calories - low in other values.
Sardines, canned in oil and drained	3 oz.	31	4	1	10	0	46	25	18	81	180	8	Rich in protein, minerals, & a desirable type of fat.
Sauerkraut	1/2 cup (2.6 oz.)	1	1	2	3	16	3	4	0	1	15	32	Fine for modern low calorie diets.
Sausage: Bologna	2 slices 4" diam. (2 oz.)	10	0	6	7	0	1	10	60	140	172	2	High in fat.
Frankfurter or hot dog	1 frankfurter (1.8 oz.)	9	0	5	6	0	1	8	54	126	155	2	Note high amount of fat.
Frankfurter or hot dog with bun	One (dog 1.8 oz., bun 1.7 oz.)	16	0	7	8	0	3	12	63	144	315	2	
Pork sausage, cooked	2 oz.	13	0	7	8	0	1	13	45	130	170	3	High in fat calories.
Vienna sausage, canned	3 oz.	19	0	5	8	0	1	20	57	126	183	3	
Scallops, cooked	3 oz.	30	0	3	8	0	4	25	1	1	109	8	Top quality protein with practically no fat.
Shad, baked	3 oz.	29	0	7	12	0	2	5	18	90	170	2	
Sherbet	1/2 cup (3.4 oz.)	2	1	1	4	0	6	1	0	0	118	2	
Sherry wine, dry	3 oz. glass	0	0	0	0	0	0	0	0	0	124	0	
Shredded wheat cereal	1 oz.	4	0	4	2	0	1	10	1	9	100	3	
Shrimp, canned	3 oz.	33	1	1	2	0	12	26	2	9	110	6	High in protein - low in fat.
Sirloin steak: Broiled	3 oz.	29	0	3	9	0	1	25	117	243	330	2	74% of the calories are from fat.
Broiled (fat trimmed)	3 oz.	37	0	4	11	0	1	31	26	51	165	3	Notice the large drop in fat calories when trimmed.
Syrup	1 tablespoon (0.7 oz.)	0	0	0	0	0	1	8	0	0	55	3	

HEALTH-BUILDING VALUES OF FOODS

FOOD	AMOUNT	PROTEIN	Vitamin A	Vitamin B₁	Vitamin B₂	Vitamin C	Calcium	Iron	Saturated Fat Calories	Total Fat Calories (Both saturated and unsaturated)	TOTAL CALORIES (From protein, fat, and carbohydrate)	V-M INDEX	REMARKS (The Vitamin-Mineral Index is shown at left. The higher the Index number, the more vitamins and minerals per calorie of food.)
		% OF DAILY ALLOWANCE											
Snap beans: Green, cooked fast, little water	1/2 cup (2.2 oz.)	1	8	3	3	12	3	4	0	1	14	39	Fine for reducing diets.
Green, cooked slowly, much water	1/2 cup (2.2 oz.)	1	8	2	3	8	3	4	0	1	14	33	Note how overcooking can reduce vitamin C.
Green, canned	1/2 cup (4.2 oz.)	1	10	2	3	6	4	16	0	1	22	31	Note lower vitamin A content of yellow beans.
Wax or yellow, canned	1/2 cup (4.2 oz.)	1	2	2	3	6	4	16	0	1	22	25	
Soda crackers	2 crackers 2-1/2" sq. (0.4 oz.)	1	0	1	1	0	0	1	4	9	45	1	
Soup: Barley soup	1 cup (8 fl. oz.)	9	1	1	3	0	10	2	9	36	115	2	
Bean soup	1 cup (8 fl. oz.)	11	0	6	6	0	12	28	18	45	190	5	
Beef soup	1 cup (8 fl. oz.)	9	0	0	0	0	2	5	18	36	100	1	
Bouillon	1 cup (8 fl. oz.)	3	0	0	3	0	0	0	0	0	10	22	Excellent for low calorie meals.
Chicken soup	1 cup (8 fl. oz.)	6	0	1	7	0	2	5	0	18	75	3	
Clam chowder	1 cup (8 fl. oz.)	7	0	0	0	0	4	36	2	18	85	8	
Cream soup such as asparagus, celery, mushroom	1 cup (8 fl. oz.)	10	4	3	11	0	27	5	63	108	200	4	
Noodle soup	1 cup (8 fl. oz.)	9	1	1	3	0	10	2	9	36	115	2	
Oyster stew with milk	1 cup w/3 to 4 oysters (8 fl. oz.)	16	13	8	22	0	34	33	22	108	200	9	
Pea soup	1 cup (8 fl. oz.)	9	9	1	4	7	4	15	9	18	140	6	
Rice soup	1 cup (8 fl. oz.)	9	1	1	3	0	10	2	9	36	115	2	
Tomato soup	1 cup (8 fl. oz.)	6	25	3	6	13	3	8	9	18	90	11	
Vegetable soup	1 cup (8 fl. oz.)	6	11	3	4	11	4	9	9	18	80	6	
Soybeans: Green, cooked	1/2 cup (2.8 oz.)	11	11	16	6	18	4	20	7	37	94	14	Contains complete protein - high in desirable linoleic acid.
Dried, cooked	1 cup (2.8 oz.)	16	1	14	6	0	9	26	11	53	107	9	
Soybean curd	1 cake 2-3/4"x2-1/2"x1" (4.2 oz.)	12	2	4	3	0	15	18	7	44	85	8	Use this to add top quality inexpensive protein to recipes.
Soybean flour	1 cup (3.1 oz.)	53	2	45	17	0	27	114	8	51	232	15	May be used by those who are allergic to milk - low in calcium.
Soybean milk (without enrichment)	1 cup (8 fl. oz.)	11	0	12	6	0	6	16	6	31	76	9	
Soybean oil	1 tablespoon (1/2 oz.)	0	0	0	0	0	0	0	18	125	125	0	High in helpful linoleic fat.
Soybean sprouts	1/2 cup (1.9 oz.)	5	2	8	6	9	3	6	2	4	25	23	A delicious food for modern low calorie meals.
Spaghetti: Enriched	1/2 cup ready to eat (2.5 oz.)	4	0	6	3	1	1	6	2	4	78	3	
With meat sauce	1/2 cup (4.4 oz.)	9	7	2	3	2	2	10	14	45	142	4	
With tomato sauce and cheese	1/2 cup (4.4 oz.)	4	8	2	2	10	3	5	9	22	105	5	
Spinach: Fresh, cooked	1/2 cup (3.2 oz.)	4	212	4	10	36	18	18	0	4	23	203	Like most greens, spinach is rich in vitamins A and C.
Canned	1/2 cup (3.2 oz.)	4	137	1	6	17	16	18	0	4	23	130	
Sponge cake	2" sector of 8" diam. cake (1.4 oz.)	2	4	2	3	0	2	6	0	18	115	2	
Sprouts: Mung bean sprouts	1/2 cup (1.6 oz.)	2	0	2	2	9	2	4	0	1	10	32	A crunchy addition to salads - delicious when steamed.
Soybean sprouts	1/2 cup (1.9 oz.)	5	2	8	6	9	3	6	1	4	25	23	A delicious food for modern low calorie meals.
Squash: Summer squash, cooked & diced	1/2 cup (3.7 oz.)	1	6	2	4	15	2	4	0	1	17	32	Excellent for modern low calorie meals.
Winter squash, baked and mashed	1/2 cup (3.6 oz.)	3	127	3	9	9	3	8	0	4	48	55	High in vitamin A.

HEALTH-BUILDING VALUES OF FOODS

FOOD	AMOUNT	PROTEIN	Vitamin A	Vitamin B_1	Vitamin B_2	Vitamin C	Calcium	Iron	Saturated Fat Calories	Total Fat Calories (Both saturated and unsaturated)	TOTAL CALORIES (From protein, fat, and carbohydrate)	V-M INDEX	REMARKS (The Vitamin-Mineral Index is shown at left. The higher the Index number, the more vitamins and minerals per calorie of food.)
Starch such as arrowroot, cornstarch, etc.	1 tablespoon (0.3 oz.)	0	0	0	0	0	0	0	0	2	30	0	
Steak cooked: Fatty cut such as sirloin	3 oz.	29	1	3	9	0	1	25	117	243	330	2	74% of the calories are from fat.
Fatty cut (outside fat trimmed)	3 oz.	37	0	4	11	0	1	31	26	51	165	5	Notice the large drop in fat calories when trimmed.
Lean cut such as round	3 oz.	34	0	4	11	0	1	30	54	117	220	3	Leaner meats contain more protein.
Lean cut (outside fat trimmed)	3 oz.	39	0	4	11	0	1	32	22	44	160	5	Note drop in saturated fat calories.
Stew, beef and vegetable	1 cup (8 fl. oz.)	21	51	8	10	19	4	28	45	90	185	11	
Strawberries	1/2 cup (2.6 oz.)	1	1	1	3	58	2	8	0	4	27	45	High in vitamin C - low in calories.
Sugar: Brown	1 tablespoon (1/2 oz.)	0	0	0	0	0	1	4	0	0	50	2	
Powdered sugar	1 tablespoon (0.3 oz.)	0	0	0	0	0	0	0	0	0	30	0	
White sugar, granulated	1 level teaspoon (0.1 oz.)	0	0	0	0	0	0	0	0	0	17	0	
White sugar, Dextra-type, enriched	1 level tablespoon (0.4 oz.)	0	0	0	0	0	0	0	0	0	50	0	Empty calories without vitamins or minerals.
	1 lump (0.2 oz.)	0	0	0	0	0	0	0	0	0	25	0	
Surinam cherry	1 tablespoon (0.4 oz.)	0	1	8	2	40	0	4	0	0	50	7	Good for vitamins A and C.
Sweet potato: Peeled after baking	3.5 oz.	3	30	6	4	32	6	10	0	4	51	25	
Peeled after boiling	1 sweet potato (5.2 oz.)	3	232	8	5	33	6	10	1	9	170	29	Loaded with vitamin A - good in other vitamins & minerals.
Candied	1 sweet potato (6.2 oz.)	3	221	6	4	23	8	16	18	54	295	16	
Canned	1/2 cup (3.8 oz.)	3	171	4	2	20	3	8	0	1	118	29	
Sweet roll	1 roll (1.5 oz.)	6	1	2	3	0	5	3	9	36	135	2	
Swiss cheese	1 oz.	10	6	1	3	0	34	3	36	72	105	7	Note saturated fat calories.
Swordfish, broiled w/butter or margarine	3 oz.	34	35	2	2	0	3	11	9	45	150	6	
Syrup	1 tablespoon (0.7 oz.)	1	0	0	0	0	3	8	0	0	55	3	
Tangerine, fresh	1 tangerine 2-1/2" diam. (4 oz.)	1	7	3	1	35	4	3	0	2	40	22	Good source of vitamin C.
Tangerine juice: Canned, unsweetened	1/2 cup (4 fl. oz.)	1	10	4	1	37	3	2	0	1	52	18	
Juice made from frozen concentrate	1/2 cup ready to drink (4 fl. oz.)	1	10	4	1	45	3	2	1	1	58	19	
Tapioca, dry, uncooked	1 tablespoon (0.4 oz.)	0	0	0	0	0	0	1	0	2	35	0	
Tea, without sugar or cream	1 cup (8 fl. oz.)	0	0	0	0	0	0	0	0	0	0	0	
Thousand Island salad dressing	1 tablespoon (1/2 oz.)	0	1	0	0	3	0	0	9	72	75	1	High in linoleic fat.
Tom Collins cocktail	1 cocktail	0	0	2	0	28	1	0	0	0	182	0	
Tomato: Fresh	1 medium tomato (5.3 oz.)	3	33	5	3	47	2	9	0	2	30	55	A good source of vitamins A & C - low in calories.
Canned or cooked	1/2 cup (4.3 oz.)	1	25	4	2	27	2	8	0	1	23	49	
Tomato juice	1/2 cup (4 fl. oz.)	1	25	4	2	25	1	5	0	1	25	41	A wholesome drink high in A and C.
Tomato catsup	1 tablespoon (0.6 oz.)	0	6	1	1	3	0	1	0	2	15	13	
Tomato soup	1 cup (8 fl. oz.)	3	25	1	6	13	3	10	2	18	90	11	
Tongue, beef, simmered	3 oz.	26	0	2	14	0	1	25	63	126	205	3	
Tortillas	1 tortilla 5" diam. (0.7 oz.)	2	1	2	1	0	3	4	0	5	50	4	
Tuna, canned in oil and drained	3 oz.	36	1	2	6	0	1	12	18	63	170	2	One of the few foods with a worthwhile amt. of vit. D.

HEALTH-BUILDING VALUES OF FOODS

FOOD	AMOUNT	PROTEIN	Vitamin A	Vitamin B_1	Vitamin B_2	Vitamin C	Calcium	Iron	Saturated Fat Calories	Total Fat Calories (Both saturated and unsaturated)	TOTAL CALORIES (From protein, fat, and carbohydrate)	V-M INDEX	REMARKS (The Vitamin-Mineral Index is shown at left. The higher the Index number, the more vitamins and minerals per calorie of food.)
					% OF DAILY ALLOWANCE								
Turkey, medium fat, cooked	1 piece without bone (3 oz.)	39	0	6	10	0	4	52	21	73	184	7	
Turkey potpie	1 pie 4 1/2" diam. (8 oz.)	24	37	4	8	0	5	16	72	252	485	2	
Turnips, cooked and diced	1/2 cup (2.7 oz.)	1	0	2	0	19	4	4	0	1	20	26	
Turnip greens: Cooked, little water, short time	1/2 cup (2.6 oz.)	3	154	3	16	58	24	18	0	4	22	207	High in vitamins A and C - very low in calories.
Cooked, much water, long time	1/2 cup (2.6 oz.)	3	154	2	14	43	24	18	0	4	22	193	Prolonged cooking reduces vitamin C.
Canned	1/2 cup (4.1 oz.)	2	102	1	6	30	14	18	0	4	20	143	
Veal cutlet, broiled	Without bone (3 oz.)	33	0	4	12	0	1	27	36	81	185	4	
Veal roast, cooked	3 oz.	33	0	7	14	0	0	29	63	126	305	3	
Vegetable oil: Corn oil	1 tablespoon (1/2 oz.)	0	0	0	0	0	0	0	18	125	125	0	Rich in desirable unsaturated linoleic fat.
Cottonseed oil	1 tablespoon (1/2 oz.)	0	0	0	0	0	0	0	18	125	125	0	Rich in desirable unsaturated linoleic fat.
Olive oil	1 tablespoon (1/2 oz.)	0	0	0	0	0	0	0	18	125	125	0	Rich in unsaturated fat though low in linoleic fat.
Soybean oil	1 tablespoon (1/2 oz.)	0	0	0	0	0	0	0	9	125	125	0	High in helpful linoleic fat.
Vegetable soup	1 cup (8 fl. oz.)	6	0	3	4	11	4	8	0	18	80	6	
Vermouth	3 oz. glass	0	0	0	0	0	0	0	0	0	150	0	More empty calories.
Vienna sausage, canned	3 oz.	19	6	5	6	0	1	20	57	126	183	3	High in fat calories.
Vinegar	1 tablespoon (1/2 oz.)	0	0	0	0	0	0	1	0	0	2	8	
Vodka, 100 proof	1 jigger (1-1/2 oz.)	0	0	0	0	0	0	0	0	0	126	0	Guaranteed to contain no vitamins or minerals.
Waffle, enriched flour	1 waffle 4-1/2"x5-1/2" (2.6 oz.)	11	0	9	12	0	16	14	27	81	240	4	High in linoleic fat.
Walnuts: Black walnuts	1 tablespoon chopped (0.3 oz.)	2	0	1	1	0	0	5	2	42	49	2	An excellent source of desirable linoleic fat.
English walnuts	1 tablespoon chopped (0.3 oz.)	1	0	2	1	0	1	2	2	45	50	2	A good source of vitamins A & C - very few calories.
Water cress	1 oz.	3	27	1	12	29	7	6	0	0	5	240	Rich in vitamins A and C.
Watermelon	1 medium slice (2 lbs. with rind)	2	51	12	3	35	4	9	1	0	120	17	Excellent for modern low calorie meals and reducing diets.
Wax beans, canned	1/2 cup (4.2 oz.)	6	2	2	3	6	1	16	0	1	22	25	
Wheat cereals: Puffed wheat	1 oz.	1	0	10	3	0	1	12	0	2	100	4	
Puffed wheat, presweetened	1 oz.	4	0	8	1	0	1	5	0	2	105	2	
Rolled wheat, cooked	1/2 cup (4.2 oz.)	4	0	5	2	0	2	4	0	4	88	3	
Shredded wheat	1 oz.	4	0	4	2	0	2	10	1	9	100	3	
Wheat and malted barley cereal	1 oz.	4	0	8	3	0	2	10	1	2	105	4	
Wheat flakes	1 oz.	4	0	10	3	0	2	10	0	2	100	5	
Wheat germ cereal	1/2 cup stirred (1.2 oz.)	12	0	43	15	0	4	28	4	32	123	12	By far the most nutritious cereal - contains complete protein.
Whipped cream: From medium cream	2 tablespoons (1/2 oz.)	0	4	0	1	0	2	0	24	44	45	3	High in saturated fat.
Whipped from heavy cream	2 tablespoons (1/2 oz.)	0	5	0	1	0	1	0	29	52	55	2	Runs up your fat total.
Whiskey: 86 proof	1 jigger (1-1/2 oz.)	0	0	0	0	0	0	0	0	0	108	0	Loaded with empty calories.
100 proof	1 jigger (1-1/2 oz.)	0	0	0	0	0	0	0	0	0	126	0	

HEALTH-BUILDING VALUES OF FOODS

FOOD	AMOUNT	% OF DAILY ALLOWANCE							Saturated Fat Calories	Total Fat Calories (Both saturated and unsaturated)	TOTAL CALORIES (From protein, fat, and carbohydrate)	V-M INDEX	REMARKS (The Vitamin-Mineral Index is shown at left. The higher the Index number, the more vitamins and minerals per calorie of food.)
		PROTEIN	Vitamin A	Vitamin B_1	Vitamin B_2	Vitamin C	Calcium	Iron					
White bread, enriched	1 slice (0.8 oz.)	3	0	4	3	0	2	6	4	9	60	4	
White sauce	1 tablespoon (0.6 oz.)	1	2	0	1	0	2	0	10	18	27	3	
Whole wheat bread	1 slice (0.8 oz.)	3	0	4	3	0	3	5	4	9	55	5	This is the most nutritious bread.
Wieners	1 wiener or frankfurter (1.8 oz.)	9	0	5	6	0	0	8	54	126	155	2	Note high amount of fat.
Wild rice, cooked	1/2 cup (2.4 oz.)	7	0	8	13	0	1	0	0	2	135	3	
Wine: Kosher	4 oz. glass	0	0	0	0	0	0	0	0	0	127	0	
Sherry, dry	3 oz. glass	0	0	0	0	0	0	0	0	2	124	0	
Yeast: Baker's cake yeast	1 oz.	4	0	12	26	0	1	14	0	2	25	35	A live yeast for cooking or baking only.
Baker's dry live yeast	1 oz.	14	0	41	85	0	2	46	0	2	80	36	Live yeast - use only for cooking or baking.
Dried Brewer's yeast	1 tablespoon (0.3 oz.)	4	0	78	19	0	2	14	0	2	25	75	Add to fruit or veg. juice for improved nutrition.
Special Torula food yeast	1 tablespoon (0.3 oz.)	6	0	125	111	0	10	15	1	5	30	145	The best source of B complex vitamins.
Yogurt, commercial	1/2 cup (4 fl. oz.)	6	2	3	12	1	18	1	9	18	60	10	A gourmet food with the benefits of milk.

NUTRITION ANALYSIS FORM

Name: _____ Date: _____

| FOOD | AMOUNT | % OF DAILY ALLOWANCE | | | | | | | Saturated Fat Calories | Total Fat Calories (Both saturated and unsaturated) | TOTAL CALORIES (From protein, fat, and carbohydrate) |
		PROTEIN	Vitamin A	Vitamin B_1	Vitamin B_2	Vitamin C	Calcium	Iron			
DAILY TOTALS		%	%	%	%	%	%	%			

DIRECTIONS:
1. List on a separate line each food you ate in a typical day.
2. Estimate about how much you ate of each food. Write this amount in the second column.
3. Find each food in the Food Table and copy figures for the various nutrients into the proper columns.
4. If you ate half the amount shown in the Food Table, cut the various figures in half. If you ate double the quantity, then double each figure before writing it on this form, etc.
5. If you ate a prepared food not shown in the Food Table, list on a separate line each of the major ingredients in your portion of the recipe. Then look them up in the Food Table as you would for other foods.
6. If you used a food that is not shown in the Food Table, substitute figures for a food that is most like the one you ate.
7. Add all columns to get your daily intake of the various nutrients.

NUTRITION ANALYSIS FORM

Name: _____ Date: _____

FOOD	AMOUNT	PROTEIN	Vitamin A	Vitamin B₁	Vitamin B₂	Vitamin C	Calcium	Iron	Saturated Fat Calories	Total Fat Calories (Both saturated and unsaturated)	TOTAL CALORIES (From protein, fat, and carbohydrate)
DAILY TOTALS		%	%	%	%	%	%	%			

% OF DAILY ALLOWANCE (spanning Protein through Iron columns)

DIRECTIONS:
1. List on a separate line each food you ate in a typical day.
2. Estimate about how much you ate of each food. Write this amount in the second column.
3. Find each food in the Food Table and copy figures for the various nutrients into the proper columns.
4. If you ate half the amount shown in the Food Table, cut the various figures in half. If you ate double the quantity, then double each figure before writing it on this form, etc.
5. If you ate a prepared food not shown in the Food Table, list on a separate line each of the major ingredients in your portion of the recipe. Then look them up in the Food Table as you would for other foods.
6. If you used a food that is not shown in the Food Table, substitute figures for a food that is most like the one you ate.
7. Add all columns to get your daily intake of the various nutrients.

NUTRITION ANALYSIS FORM

Name: _____   Date: _____

FOOD	AMOUNT	% OF DAILY ALLOWANCE							Saturated Fat Calories	Total Fat Calories (Both saturated and unsaturated)	TOTAL CALORIES (From protein, fat, and carbohydrate)
		PROTEIN	Vitamin A	Vitamin B₁	Vitamin B₂	Vitamin C	Calcium	Iron			
DAILY TOTALS		%	%	%	%	%	%	%			

DIRECTIONS:
1. List on a separate line each food you ate in a typical day.
2. Estimate about how much you ate of each food. Write this amount in the second column.
3. Find each food in the Food Table and copy figures for the various nutrients into the proper columns.
4. If you ate half the amount shown in the Food Table, cut the various figures in half. If you ate double the quantity, then double each figure before writing it on this form, etc.
5. If you ate a prepared food not shown in the Food Table, list on a separate line each of the major ingredients in your portion of the recipe. Then look them up in the Food Table as you would for other foods.
6. If you used a food that is not shown in the Food Table, substitute figures for a food that is most like the one you ate.
7. Add all columns to get your daily intake of the various nutrients.

NUTRITION ANALYSIS FORM

Name: _____ Date: _____

| FOOD | AMOUNT | % OF DAILY ALLOWANCE | | | | | | | Saturated Fat Calories | Total Fat Calories (Both saturated and unsaturated) | TOTAL CALORIES (From protein, fat, and carbohydrate) |
		PROTEIN	Vitamin A	Vitamin B₁	Vitamin B₂	Vitamin C	Calcium	Iron			
DAILY TOTALS		%	%	%	%	%	%	%			

DIRECTIONS:
1. List on a separate line each food you ate in a typical day.
2. Estimate about how much you ate of each food. Write this amount in the second column.
3. Find each food in the Food Table and copy figures for the various nutrients into the proper columns.
4. If you ate half the amount shown in the Food Table, cut the various figures in half. If you ate double the quantity, then double each figure before writing it on this form, etc.
5. If you ate a prepared food not shown in the Food Table, list on a separate line each of the major ingredients in your portion of the recipe. Then look them up in the Food Table as you would for other foods.
6. If you used a food that is not shown in the Food Table, substitute figures for a food that is most like the one you ate.
7. Add all columns to get your daily intake of the various nutrients.

NUTRITION ANALYSIS FORM

Name: _____ Date: _____

| FOOD | AMOUNT | % OF DAILY ALLOWANCE | | | | | | | Saturated Fat Calories | Total Fat Calories (Both saturated and unsaturated) | TOTAL CALORIES (From protein, fat, and carbohydrate) |
		PROTEIN	Vitamin A	Vitamin B$_1$	Vitamin B$_2$	Vitamin C	Calcium	Iron			
DAILY TOTALS		%	%	%	%	%	%	%			

DIRECTIONS:
1. List on a separate line each food you ate in a typical day.
2. Estimate about how much you ate of each food. Write this amount in the second column.
3. Find each food in the Food Table and copy figures for the various nutrients into the proper columns.
4. If you ate half the amount shown in the Food Table, cut the various figures in half. If you ate double the quantity, then double each figure before writing it on this form, etc.
5. If you ate a prepared food not shown in the Food Table, list on a separate line each of the major ingredients in your portion of the recipe. Then look them up in the Food Table as you would for other foods.
6. If you used a food that is not shown in the Food Table, substitute figures for a food that is most like the one you ate.
7. Add all columns to get your daily intake of the various nutrients.

NUTRITION ANALYSIS FORM

Name: _____ Date: _____

FOOD	AMOUNT	% OF DAILY ALLOWANCE							Saturated Fat Calories	Total Fat Calories (Both saturated and unsaturated)	TOTAL CALORIES (From protein, fat, and carbohydrate)
		PROTEIN	Vitamin A	Vitamin B$_1$	Vitamin B$_2$	Vitamin C	Calcium	Iron			
DAILY TOTALS		%	%	%	%	%	%	%			

DIRECTIONS:
1. List on a separate line each food you ate in a typical day.
2. Estimate about how much you ate of each food. Write this amount in the second column.
3. Find each food in the Food Table and copy figures for the various nutrients into the proper columns.
4. If you ate half the amount shown in the Food Table, cut the various figures in half. If you ate double the quantity, then double each figure before writing it on this form, etc.
5. If you ate a prepared food not shown in the Food Table, list on a separate line each of the major ingredients in your portion of the recipe. Then look them up in the Food Table as you would for other foods.
6. If you used a food that is not shown in the Food Table, substitute figures for a food that is most like the one you ate.
7. Add all columns to get your daily intake of the various nutrients

NUTRITION ANALYSIS FORM

Name: _____ Date: _____

| FOOD | AMOUNT | % OF DAILY ALLOWANCE | | | | | | | Saturated Fat Calories | Total Fat Calories (Both saturated and unsaturated) | TOTAL CALORIES (From protein, fat, and carbohydrate) |
		PROTEIN	Vitamin A	Vitamin B₁	Vitamin B₂	Vitamin C	Calcium	Iron			
DAILY TOTALS		%	%	%	%	%	%	%			

DIRECTIONS:
1. List on a separate line each food you ate in a typical day.
2. Estimate about how much you ate of each food. Write this amount in the second column.
3. Find each food in the Food Table and copy figures for the various nutrients into the proper columns.
4. If you ate half the amount shown in the Food Table, cut the various figures in half. If you ate double the quantity, then double each figure before writing it on this form, etc.
5. If you ate a prepared food not shown in the Food Table, list on a separate line each of the major ingredients in your portion of the recipe. Then look them up in the Food Table as you would for other foods.
6. If you used a food that is not shown in the Food Table, substitute figures for a food that is most like the one you ate.
7. Add all columns to get your daily intake of the various nutrients.

NUTRITION ANALYSIS FORM

Name: ______________________________ **Date:** ______________

FOOD	AMOUNT	% OF DAILY ALLOWANCE							Saturated Fat Calories	Total Fat Calories (Both saturated and unsaturated)	TOTAL CALORIES (From protein, fat, and carbohydrate)
		PROTEIN	Vitamin A	Vitamin B_1	Vitamin B_2	Vitamin C	Calcium	Iron			
	DAILY TOTALS	%	%	%	%	%	%	%			

DIRECTIONS:

1. List on a separate line each food you ate in a typical day.
2. Estimate about how much you ate of each food. Write this amount in the second column.
3. Find each food in the Food Table and copy figures for the various nutrients into the proper columns.
4. If you ate half the amount shown in the Food Table, cut the various figures in half. If you ate double the quantity, then double each figure before writing it on this form, etc.
5. If you ate a prepared food not shown in the Food Table, list on a separate line each of the major ingredients in your portion of the recipe. Then look them up in the Food Table as you would for other foods.
6. If you used a food that is not shown in the Food Table, substitute figures for a food that is most like the one you ate.
7. Add all columns to get your daily intake of the various nutrients.

NUTRITION ANALYSIS FORM

Name: ______________________________ **Date:** ______________

FOOD	AMOUNT	% OF DAILY ALLOWANCE							Saturated Fat Calories	Total Fat Calories (Both saturated and unsaturated)	TOTAL CALORIES (From protein, fat, and carbohydrate)
		PROTEIN	Vitamin A	Vitamin B_1	Vitamin B_2	Vitamin C	Calcium	Iron			
	DAILY TOTALS	%	%	%	%	%	%	%			

DIRECTIONS:

1. List on a separate line each food you ate in a typical day.
2. Estimate about how much you ate of each food. Write this amount in the second column.
3. Find each food in the Food Table and copy figures for the various nutrients into the proper columns.
4. If you ate half the amount shown in the Food Table, cut the various figures in half. If you ate double the quantity, then double each figure before writing it on this form, etc.
5. If you ate a prepared food not shown in the Food Table, list on a separate line each of the major ingredients in your portion of the recipe. Then look them up in the Food Table as you would for other foods.
6. If you used a food that is not shown in the Food Table, substitute figures for a food that is most like the one you ate.
7. Add all columns to get your daily intake of the various nutrients.

NUTRITION ANALYSIS FORM

Name: ______________________________ Date: ______________

FOOD	AMOUNT	% OF DAILY ALLOWANCE							Saturated Fat Calories	Total Fat Calories (Both saturated and unsaturated)	TOTAL CALORIES (From protein, fat, and carbohydrate)
		PROTEIN	Vitamin A	Vitamin B_1	Vitamin B_2	Vitamin C	Calcium	Iron			
	DAILY TOTALS	%	%	%	%	%	%	%			

DIRECTIONS:

1. List on a separate line each food you ate in a typical day.
2. Estimate about how much you ate of each food. Write this amount in the second column.
3. Find each food in the Food Table and copy figures for the various nutrients into the proper columns.
4. If you ate half the amount shown in the Food Table, cut the various figures in half. If you ate double the quantity, then double each figure before writing it on this form, etc.
5. If you ate a prepared food not shown in the Food Table, list on a separate line each of the major ingredients in your portion of the recipe. Then look them up in the Food Table as you would for other foods.
6. If you used a food that is not shown in the Food Table, substitute figures for a food that is most like the one you ate.
7. Add all columns to get your daily intake of the various nutrients.

NUTRITION ANALYSIS FORM

Name: _____ Date: _____

| FOOD | AMOUNT | % OF DAILY ALLOWANCE | | | | | | | Saturated Fat Calories | Total Fat Calories (Both saturated and unsaturated) | TOTAL CALORIES (From protein, fat, and carbohydrate) |
		PROTEIN	Vitamin A	Vitamin B₁	Vitamin B₂	Vitamin C	Calcium	Iron			
DAILY TOTALS		%	%	%	%	%	%	%			

DIRECTIONS:
1. List on a separate line each food you ate in a typical day.
2. Estimate about how much you ate of each food. Write this amount in the second column.
3. Find each food in the Food Table and copy figures for the various nutrients into the proper columns.
4. If you ate half the amount shown in the Food Table, cut the various figures in half. If you ate double the quantity, then double each figure before writing it on this form, etc.
5. If you ate a prepared food not shown in the Food Table, list on a separate line each of the major ingredients in your portion of the recipe. Then look them up in the Food Table as you would for other foods.
6. If you used a food that is not shown in the Food Table, substitute figures for a food that is most like the one you ate.
7. Add all columns to get your daily intake of the various nutrients.

NUTRITION ANALYSIS FORM

Name: _____ Date: _____

| FOOD | AMOUNT | % OF DAILY ALLOWANCE | | | | | | | Saturated Fat Calories | Total Fat Calories (Both saturated and unsaturated) | TOTAL CALORIES (From protein, fat, and carbohydrate) |
		PROTEIN	Vitamin A	Vitamin B₁	Vitamin B₂	Vitamin C	Calcium	Iron			
DAILY TOTALS		%	%	%	%	%	%	%			

DIRECTIONS:
1. List on a separate line each food you ate in a typical day.
2. Estimate about how much you ate of each food. Write this amount in the second column.
3. Find each food in the Food Table and copy figures for the various nutrients into the proper columns.
4. If you ate half the amount shown in the Food Table, cut the various figures in half. If you ate double the quantity, then double each figure before writing it on this form, etc.
5. If you ate a prepared food not shown in the Food Table, list on a separate line each of the major ingredients in your portion of the recipe. Then look them up in the Food Table as you would for other foods.
6. If you used a food that is not shown in the Food Table, substitute figures for a food that is most like the one you ate.
7. Add all columns to get your daily intake of the various nutrients.

THE CORNUCOPIA INSTITUTE

The Cornucopia Institute is located on a 115 acre campus in St. Mary, Kentucky. The Institute is dedicated to teaching the "Science of Happiness." It offers courses ranging from a weekend to four years. The teachings at the Institute are based on the *Handbook to Higher Consciousness* by Ken Keyes, Jr. The *Handbook* presents a method whereby one can live a continuously enjoyable and fulfilling life—regardless of the day-to-day circumstances presented by the world in which we live.

If you would like to improve your life and environment through the Science of Happiness, please inquire about our non-profit programs by writing for a brochure and catalog of coming events. We will send you information on available literature, cassette recordings, phonograph records, posters, and out-of-state workshops that are scheduled in other parts of the country. Letters should be addressed to the Cornucopia Institute, St. Mary, Kentucky 40063.

Other books by Ken Keyes, Jr.

Handbook to Higher Consciousness
by Ken Keyes, Jr.
5½ x 8½", perfect bound, $2.95; hardbound edition, $4.95
This book presents the "science of happiness" in practical, everyday terms that you can apply to your own life. It shows you how you can be perceptive, loving, happy, and fulfilled all of the time—in spite of all of the conditions in your life that you are now sure are keeping you from feeling secure and happy. Countless people have experienced that their lives have changed dramatically from the time they began to apply the practical methods explained in the Handbook to Higher Consciousness.

How to Make Your Life Work or Why Aren't You Happy?
by Ken Keyes, Jr., and Bruce Burkan
5½ x 8½", perfect bound, $2.00
This book is fun to read! Every other page is a delightful, to-the-point cartoon that adds meaning to the timely message. You may find that this simple, enjoyable book gives you the one thing you've been missing to enable your life to be really great!

Taming Your Mind
by Ken Keyes, Jr.
5½x 8½", clothbound, $4.95
This enjoyable book (which has been in print for 25 years) shows you how to use your mind more effectively. It contains about 80 full-page drawings by the famous illustrator, Ted Key. It is written in a deeply effective but entertaining style. It was previously published under the title How To Develop Your Thinking Ability. It was adopted by two book clubs and has sold over 100,000 copies. Available through bookstores or from the Cornucopia Institute, St. Mary, Kentucky 40063. Please enclose 25¢ per book for postage and packaging.

252